To Dr. Ram
with my very best
wishes for your
health and
happiness.

Mousatapha

Moustafa Ahmed, writer and journalist, born in Egypt, received his higher education in Egypt and Britain. Read, English Literature, Phonetics, International Affairs, Media, and Anthropology. He was a foreign correspondent based in the UK for an Egyptian newspaper and a magazine. He published a new magazine 'The Politician' in 1989, and was its editor until it ceased publication in 1995 because of his illness. Author of many articles and books, published in both Arabic and English. He is also a co-author of many researches on international affairs.

Professor G M Dusheiko, MB BCh, FCP (SA) FRCP FRCP (Edin.), Professor of medicine and honorary consultant at the Royal Free and University College Medical School, London, UK. Published many research articles on Pathogenesis, immune responsiveness and therapy of chronic hepatitis.

SURVIVING LIVER DISEASES
LIFE WITH A LIVER TRANSPLANT

SURVIVING LIVER DISEASES

LIFE WITH A LIVER TRANSPLANT

Moustafa Ahmed

Foreword by
Professor
G. M. Dusheiko, MB BCh, FCP(SA) FRCP FRCP (Edin)

MegaZette Press
London, UK.

To my daughter Sarah and my family

Copyright 1999 by Moustafa Ahmed

First published in 1999 in the United Kingdom
by MegaZette Press

All rights reserved. No part of this book may be reproduced,
stored in a retrieval system, or transmitted, in any form or
by any means without the prior written permission of the
author and the publisher of this book,
nor be otherwise circulated in any form of binding or cover
other than that in which it is published and without a
similar condition being imposed on the subsequent
purchaser.

British Library Cataloguing-in-Publication Data
A CIP catalogue record for this book is available from the
British Library

ISBN: 0-9536007-0-X

Designed by MegaZette Press
Printed in the UK

MegaZette Press
PO Box 269,
Middlesex, HA8 9HN, UK

CONTENTS

Foreword
Acknowledgements
Introduction

BOOK ONE
MY STORY

1
Early Signs 15
2
First Admission 26
3
At The Royal Free Hospital 31
4
Breaking The News 40
5
The Dentist's Chair 46
6
The Coma 51
7
The Transplantation 57
8
One Year After 66

BOOK TWO
CARING FOR YOUR LIVER

1
Facts And Figures 77
2
The Liver And Its Structure 79
3
Caring For Your Liver 82
4
Eating For A Healthy Liver 86
5
Liver Diseases 92
6
Liver Transplantation 105
7
Questions And Answers
    1- On hepatitis 112
    2- On liver Transplantation 116

Glossary 123
References

LIST OF ILLUSTRATIONS

- The Royal Free Hospital Hampstead, London
- Inside Hassall Ward, Dr. D. Patch, Dr.Sean Dixon, Sister Kate Whitfield, and Ward Manager Simone Quirin.
- British Secretary of state for Health, Mr Frank Dobson with consultant physician Dr. A. Burroughs Consultant Surgeon Mr. K. Rolles and Chief Executive Mr. M. Else.
- Rt. Hon. Mr. Frank Dobson presents Yvonne McGarry, a liver transplant coordinator with a bouquet of flowers.
- Rt. Hon. Mr. Frank Dobson presents Geraldine Amooty, a liver transplant coordinator with a bouquet of flowers.
- Rt. Hon. Mr. Frank Dobson presents Mr. Larry Davis Business manager, with a bouquet of flowers.
- Liver transplant coordinator, Linda Selves with a liver transplant patient in the outpatients clinic.
- Consultant Dr. D. Patch with a liver transplant patient, and Hassall Ward Manager, Sister Simone Quirin, and Sister Jackui Winship.
- The Author with the British Secretary of state for Health Mr. Frank Dobson and another liver transplant patient.
- Rt. Hon. Mr. F. Dobson, Dr. A. Burroughs and Mr. Rolles with a group of liver transplant patients at the celebration of 500 liver transplants.

Foreword

This is an interesting and moving account of the experience of one man of his liver transplant at the Royal Free Hospital. Moustafa gives a chronological account of the onset of his illness to the point at which he received a liver transplant, and his post-transplant experience. He also has included a non-technical section on liver diseases, viral hepatitis and liver transplantation.

His account moves from his inherent faith in nature to heal his chronic liver disease to the realisation that he had reached the point in his illness at which he needed to place his faith in liver transplantation and scientific medicine, in order to survive.

The chapters are divided, so as to lead the reader chronologically through the patient's first early signs of liver disease, his worsening clinical state, admission, the onset of hepatic encephalopathy, and transplant work-up until his liver transplant and beyond.

The author takes the reader through his alternating emotions, ranging from the depths of his despair and uncertainty to redemption and hope. The author gives a colourful description of his psychological acceptance of the transplanted liver.

He is understandably familiar with the nature of chronic hepatitis, and gives the reader a graphic account of his symptoms and illness.

The book is a reminder to physicians and surgeons of the patients' viewpoint, seen from the bedside or examination couch. His book challenges physicians and reminds them of the confusion that may still exist in the minds of patients when the physician believes that he or she has explained matters with absolute clarity.

The second part of this book includes a description in layman's language of liver physiology, with sections on diet and alcohol and descriptions of common liver diseases particularly viral hepatitis, liver transplantation, and liver transplant work up.

The author provides important information concerning the global burden of hepatitis C, and the continued high infection in many countries world-wide.

This book is at times an amusing narrative, and includes several passages of self deprecating humour, for example Mr. Moustafa's recounting of the hospital Chef serving Christmas dinner. It is written with both with humour and fortitude that will provide interest and inspiration for patients and health carers alike.

Prof. Geoffrey Dusheiko

Acknowledgements

It is difficult to recall all those who have conscientiously cared for my health at the Royal Free Hospital, and it is also impossible to thank all of them since mere words would do little to convey the quality and depth of my gratitude.

Nevertheless, certain names need to be mentioned. I am in debt to Professor G. Dusheiko, professor of medicine at the Royal Free and University College Medical School, and to all the liver transplant team at the Royal Free Hospital, in particular Mr. K. Rolles Consultant Surgeon, Dr. A. Burroughs Consultant Physician, Dr. D. Patch Consultant Physician, Dr. P. Mistry Consultant Physician, Professor N. McIntyre, Dr. J. Dooley and the Consultant Anaesthetists.

I am also very grateful to the liver transplant coordinators, Linda Selves, Geraldine Amooty, and Yvonne McGarry. I am also in debt to Simone Quirin, Hassall Ward Manager, and to all sisters and nursing staff at the Hassall Ward, Royal Free Hospital.

My deep gratitude to Dr. Zoe Pinto my GP, and to Dr. Bevan, and Dr. G. Webster, Dr. Ralph Greaves, Dr. Keshav, Mr. Rahul Kot, Dr. Mandour El-Mahdi, Dr. M. Al Wahsh, Dr. M. Sherry.

My sincere gratitude to my friends, Mr. Mohamed Al Fayed chairman of Harrods, and to H.E. Dr. Mohamed Shaker former Egyptian Ambassador to the UK, for their support.

I would like also to thank all my friends and colleagues, Mrs. A. Smith, Miss B. White, Mr. & Mrs. Al Gouhari, Mr. & Mrs A. Mossab, Mr. & Mrs. A. Hamouda, Mr. Attallah, Mr. I. Nawar, Mr. M. Al Behari, Dr. Al Sharqawi, Mr. & Mrs. Khetia, Mr. H. Sharouni.

Last but by no means least, my thanks to all members of my family.

Introduction

The main aim in writing this book is to tell my story, and to give my experience with a damaged liver as well as to provide information on liver diseases and liver transplantation. It is also to raise the alarm about the seriousness of these terrible diseases particularly, hepatitis viruses, and liver cirrhosis. Also to express my horror of the spread of hepatitis viruses around the world, and my scepticism of the way that governments, and media around the world, are dealing with these serious liver diseases.

I was inspired to write this book by a patient who was lying in a bed opposite to mine in a 4-bedded room in Hassall Ward, at the Royal Free Hospital. I was regaining consciousness and recovering from a coma, and he was recovering from a liver transplantation.

He came to my bed one evening to tell me his story with his illness. I could see from his story how much he had suffered from the complications of liver damage, and how he was saved by the liver transplantation.

He was as shocked as I was, when he was diagnosed as having a serious liver disease that he had never heard of before.

At that time I was neither sure about my recovery from liver damage, nor about giving my consent to the liver transplantation. However, I listened carefully to what he said for I was desperately in need of anyone who could give me some encouragement that would enable me to take this hard decision. A decision that could be vital and fatal.

Talking to a patient who had experienced liver transplantation was quite useful as well as an opportunity for myself to learn more about it. The experience that I would go through one day.

As a journalist, my illness provided me with an opportunity to investigate the seriousness of these diseases, and how they are spreading rapidly around the world. It is unfortunate that liver diseases are poorly understood among the majority of peoples around the world.

I was surprised when I discovered that many people do not have the slightest idea about liver diseases especially hepatitis viruses and liver cirrhosis.

My observation has led me to believe that we know and care more about the heart than any other organ in the human body. I was surprised to see that the amount of literature and publicity on caring for the liver is in short supply, whereas the amount of literature and publicity on caring for the heart and the prevention of heart disease is immense.

Take smoking for example, everyone knows that smoking causes lung cancer and heart problems, however, very few people know that smoking can be a cause of liver damage. Another example is that, we all know that alcohol can raise blood pressure, and cause coronary heart disease, nevertheless, very few people know that alcohol can cause liver damage, and liver cirrhosis.

At present, there is a publicity campaign running to legalize cannabis, and to use it as pain relief for patients who suffer from cancer. However, do we know that cannabis can seriously damage the liver?

There are many other examples that prove without doubt that we are living in the dark as far as the liver, our vital organ, is concerned.

In essence the liver serves as an engine, a refinery. Anything that we eat, drink or even smell, goes to the liver to be refined and to rid it of poisonous substances before it is transmitted to the other parts of the human body.

The human liver is a 'silent partner,' a non-complaining, 'noble organ,' that needs your care and attention to stay healthy. Unfortunately, the liver does not usually let you know when it is in trouble, and keeps working until it is completely damaged. That is why caring for the liver is not only important, but it is a must.

Any type and amount of literature and information that helps us to stay healthy is very important, for there is nothing better in life than staying healthy. However, directing all our efforts and resources, and concentrating on caring for only one organ, and neglecting other vital organs, is an undesirable attitude.

Caring for the liver has positive effects on the general health of the human body.

In the past, the liver enjoyed a good place among the people who built the ancient civilizations. Ancient Egyptians and ancient Greeks thought of the liver as the most important organ inside the human body.

In eastern cultures, the liver used to occupy an important place, as the centre of the human body.

Indeed it was the "noble organ" but at the present it is the "forgotten organ."

The word 'liver' itself derives from the verb 'to live" in English, as it does in German, with 'leber' and 'leben'. In the Arabic language they say, 'Kabid Al Hakika', (liver of the matter) which means in English 'heart of the matter'. They also say 'Kabid Al-Sama', 'Centre of the heaven or the sky'.

In spoken Egyptian Arabic they say 'Hita min Kabidi', it is translated in the English language as, 'A piece of my liver'. This phrase is used to describe some one who is very precious. However, modern Egyptians have changed it at present to be 'Hita min qalbi', 'A piece of my heart'.

It is clear that, for some reason, the liver has gradually lost its position and it has been replaced by the heart in its importance.

Jacques Cinqualbre, Professor of surgery at the University of Strasbourg Medical School says in his article, 'Symbolism of the Liver Through the Ages' that, *"However, for some reason, the liver was about to lose most or all of its luster, and would be soon denied the qualification of noble organ which was transferred to the heart. Even though being nothing more than a sophisticated pump, the heart is emotionally considered more important than any other organ including the brain."*

Few people know that the liver acts as a filter and can be badly damaged by drinking too much alcohol. Other than that they know little about the complexities and the importance of the many vital functions the liver performs.

Every year millions of people are diagnosed as having liver and gallbladder diseases, and many people die of liver disease each year. However, there are few effective treatments for most life-threatening liver diseases, except for liver transplants.

World Health Organization (WHO) has stated in its report that liver diseases are spreading rapidly in both developed and developing countries. According to a World Health Organization report, *"Hepatitis B has infected 2 billion people alive today, of whom 350 million are chronically and incurably infected with hepatitis C."*

Experts estimate that more than half of all liver diseases could be prevented if people start caring for their livers in the early days, and not wait till the liver is completely damaged.

An adequate investment in effective liver research has the potential of saving billions of pounds and preventing untold human suffering.

The government of any society must put the health of its people first, as a priority. People will produce more wealth if they are healthy. I learnt in my early school days that, illness, poverty, and ignorance, are the three main enemies that stand against the progress or the development of any society. Healthy people create a healthy society.

We need to locate more funds and resources to promote the importance of caring for the liver.

I hope that this book will help patients, as well as doctors, nurses and anyone caring for the general health of people.

This book is a reminder for all of us, to care, and to think about the liver, as a vital organ in the human body.

There are many people who are in urgent need for information that help them to learn more about the liver, and liver diseases. Unfortunately, it seems to me that there are limited resources allocated for this purpose.

In the United States of America they take liver diseases very seriously, and the Congress convenes many hearings to discuss the public threat posed by the widespread of hepatitis viruses. The most recent debate was held in march 1998.

Another example, is that, the Hepatitis Foundation International, has scheduled its annual National Hepatitis Congress and Walk on Washington in March 1999, at Georgetown University.

There is no doubt that these conferences and debates are of vital importance in making people aware of the danger of liver diseases. That is why it is essential that politicians and people who are working for the media around the world should not spare any effort in helping the public to make them aware of these facts.

Moustafa Ahmed   ***London, March, 99***

12

BOOK ONE

MY STORY

1

Early Signs

It was a dry beautiful summer day of July 1995. The sun was shining, the sky was blue and the air was fresh and pleasant. The weather was perfect, an ideal day for a summer holiday.

Looking down at the street from my bedroom window, the beautiful roses and the colourful flowers were blooming. The sounds of lawn mowers were roaring in almost every garden, and the delightful aroma of freshly cut grass was spreading through the gentle air of this lovely morning.

People were extremely happy and cheerful, broad smiles covered almost every face. They were exceptionally friendly and sociable. Expressions such as 'fine day' and 'beautiful weather' were the most common phrases one could hear.

The summer heat had melted the ice barriers of the cold winter. How much happiness sun shine brings to people! How much the weather can change our mood!

Sometimes I wonder, why people are obsessed by

the weather, complaining, praising, and generally talking so much about it. Is it because the weather concerns all of us? Is it because the weather is considered to be a suitable topic to start any serious conversation? Is it because our life is somehow dependent on it?

It is more likely that our life on earth resembles and follows the same pattern as the weather. Our birth, our death; our ups our downs; infancy, juvenility, maturity and old age. Spring, summer, autumn and winter. I am not really sure. Nothing is certain in this world.

However, there was one thing that I was positive about on that particular day. I was quite certain that I was going to stay at home for the whole day. The reason, I was feeling unwell.

I had been waiting eagerly for such a beautiful day, to be able to enjoy it to the full, but when the chance came I could not.

I was not prepared to accept that the weather was beautiful, but I was unable to move from my home to enjoy it.

I had to stay at home all day, or perhaps even for a few more days. The inability to do something that one enjoys is in itself, torture. That feeling was enough to put me off and to make me miserable on such a beautiful day.

It was impossible for me to go out, or even to work in the garden. I was worried, and anxious. Worried about what was happening and eager to know the reason.

However, the reason for staying at home on such a beautiful day, was not convincing. I found it rather funny. For not being able to put my shoes on, was a weird reason. I did not have a pair of shoes that would fit my feet! What was more, both my feet were very big, they were swollen!

When I got up that morning, I was keen to go out, but when I tried to put my shoes on, I had no other alternative but to change my mind and stay at home.

I noticed that both my feet and ankles were swollen. The reason was beyond my comprehension. At first, I could not be bothered with this nonsense or even to take any notice of it, but when I tried my shoes, I started to wonder.

The more I thought of both my feet, the more I became depressed, and worried. My wife and my daughter were surprised to see my feet in such a state.

It was not a good idea to sit down, looking at my swollen feet, guessing the causes and the reasons. I consulted a medical encyclopaedia and I looked at the causes, but what was the use of it? There are many causes of the same symptom.

It was an awful time, and I hated it. I tried to keep myself busy. I started to think about my work, and to forget about my swollen feet, but unfortunately I lost the ability to concentrate.

I had to write an article for my magazine. That was a good excuse, sufficient enough to persuade myself to stay at home happily even though I did not write one word.

Keeping myself busy, or pretending I was busy, was almost a kind of escapism. I did not like to think that I was staying at home because of my swollen feet. I promised myself, that nothing would stop me from working. But at that particular time I was confronted with the absolute truth, with reality.

Frankly, I was a very worried man, expressing my fear and my uneasiness in silence. I had to keep my anxiety to myself. My philosophy, was to share happiness, and hide anxieties. I must admit I was wrong. I learnt, although it was too late, that a healthy attitude in life, is to share anxieties, as well as happiness.

I knew I was workaholic, working day and night, and I knew I was exhausted, and what I needed was a long break. I also knew that I had to convince myself to go to see my doctor for a thorough check-up, even though I did not approve of going to see my doctor as a patient. I used to believe that the human body is capable of healing any defect by itself. Medications and their side effects could make matters worse.

I had to wait till Monday to see my doctor, and I hoped by that time both my feet would return to their normal size.

Saturday and Sunday passed slowly, and my feet were still the same, no change for the better. On Monday morning I phoned my GP, Doctor Zoe Pinto, and I made an emergency appointment to see her. The same day, in the afternoon I went to see her in the surgery.

The distance between my home and the surgery takes normally about five minutes walking, but that day it took more than fifteen minutes, and when I arrived I was breathless.

After the doctor examined me, she gave me the good news that I was eager to hear. I had nothing to worry about, but I needed to be mobile. I had to walk for at least twenty minutes a day, and to take some exercises.

I was relieved when I heard the news. It was exactly what I wanted to hear. I was listening carefully to what she said, and I took her words at face value, never questioning her. Her words were sufficient to convince me that the advice I was given was right. Her medical recommendations were sound and good, at least for me.

I started to put the blame on myself for not taking enough physical exercises, and for sitting for long hours working at my desk. However, to celebrate the news, we went out for dinner, and I bought myself a pair of large size trainers.

I began to walk for at least twenty minutes a day, and doing some exercise for another twenty minute every evening. I hoped that by doing so regularly, I would feel better and my feet would go back to its normal size. But it did not, and to my surprise, my feet became even bigger. In addition to that I started to feel pain around the upper part of my abdomen.

Two weeks later, I went to see my doctor again. I told her about the new development. Doctor Pinto examined me thoroughly, and for no apparent reason she examined my eyes, and after she finished, she asked me to make an appointment to see the nurse for a blood test, which I did.

A week later, I went to see my doctor again. At that time she had started to suspect something, "I will refer you to Edgware General Hospital in North London for an Ultrasound scan" she said. Immediately I questioned her, and to my surprise I was told, "it is just to make sure that there is nothing wrong with your liver". My liver! What is wrong with my liver? That was a big joke, certainly a mistake.

I had never expected any thing wrong with my liver. I was expecting, that she would say, the reason for feeling unwell, was the exhaustion from long working hours, or if the worse came to worse, she might have said that there was something wrong with my heart. Certainly not with my liver.

I never thought that I would suffer from my liver. I used to think that the only organ in the human body that could cause trouble was the heart.

Physically, I was feeling unwell, and I knew there was something wrong somewhere in my body, but I did not have a clue in what part of my body. My body had given me the message a long time ago, but I ignored it, or to put it more bluntly I preferred not to listen.

Working as journalist, is a twenty-four hour

occupation. I used to spend all day and part of the night working, and now I had to pay the price. But it was a heavy price.

However, I had learnt, although it was too late, to listen to my body. The feeling of being unwell is terrible enough, but going to hospital as a patient is even more frightening. I had never been to a hospital as a patient before, but now I had to.

Thinking all the way about what I was going to say or what they were going to do, let alone what they were going to tell me, was really frightening.

In hospital, I walked through a long corridor. Its walls were covered with tiles, giving the impression of an old building. The corridor led me in the direction of the ultrasound department. I sat in the waiting area for nearly ten minutes. When I was called, I went inside the consulting room and the doctor asked me to take off my shirt and to lie down on a trolley, while she was busy fixing the computer terminal to make it ready for a new patient.

I was able to see my liver on the screen, but I could not interpret the picture. After the doctor had a clear scan, I was asked to make an appointment to see my GP in one week.

A week later, I went to see my GP Doctor Pinto. Inside her room, she was sitting looking at my ultrasound report. I sat down on a chair opposite to her. She had to examine me by looking first deeply into my left eye.

I was staring at her face, watching her expression, trying to interpret what was going on her mind. In a gentle soft voice Doctor Pinto told me that my liver was not functioning well and she would refer me to Doctor Bevan a consultant in Edgware General Hospital. I asked her for more explanations. She told me that I was suffering from liver damage and I might also suffering from hepatitis C.

I might have understood what she meant by liver damage even though I did not know to what extent. What I could not understand at that time was, what she meant by hepatitis C.

My knowledge of hepatitis disease, in general, was very poor indeed, if anything at all. I asked her many questions about that disease, but she was very economical in her answers.

Doctor Pinto is a very gentle doctor, and I could understand what she felt at that moment. However, she assured me that Doctor Bevan would explain every thing to me.

I fell silent, not a word to be said, not even a comment from her either. I kept quiet for a few seconds, just looking at her, as if I was waiting for more explanation, but she did not give the answers that would satisfy my curiosity.

She realised that I was worried, and she tried hard but in vain, to stop me from worrying. She prescribed a medicine to take until I go to see Doctor Bevan in Edgware General Hospital.

I left the surgery quite convinced that I had a serious disease, but I decided not to surrender to any fear of disease. I thought that by freeing myself from some stressful burdens I would free myself from diseases.

At home I told my wife what my doctor said, she was as astonished as I was. She asked me many questions that I was unable to answer.

Sometimes ignorance is bliss. My poor knowledge of hepatitis disease, let alone hepatitis C, made me unaware about the extent of that disease. That helped me initially a great deal in easing off my worry.

I started to take the medication that my doctor prescribed to me. As a result of that medication, I lost weight and I looked well, slim and smart, even though, I did not know how the medicine worked.

I felt much better than before, and I thought that I was already recovered, without seeing Doctor Bevan. All my best suits fitted me at that time and I started to look after my health. I understood, but it was later on, that I had some fluid in my body, and the medication was actually a diuretic helping my body to get rid of that fluid. That was how I lost weight.

Making fun of the situation to ease off the pain of the harsh reality is in my view the best pain relief. I had learnt in life, that if I could not find something to laugh at, I could laugh at myself. I tried this method together with doing other things that would help me in keeping my thoughts away from the bitter reality. I was trying hard to forget the suffering of the present, and the obscurity of the future.

To pretend that things are looking bright, and to be hopeful is good, but to ignore the facts completely is an imprudent thing to do. Facts remain facts and never change. The fact was, I was seriously ill. Fatigue became somehow permanent. My face and my eyes were pale and yellow, and I could not perceive any brightness in them at all. Even after my health had improved slightly, I began to feel unwell again. I was gaining weight, and my abdomen became large and strained. My state of health was deteriorating rapidly. I understood later that all these symptoms were in fact a result of an accumulation of fluid inside my abdomen, which is medically known as 'ascetics.'

Three weeks later, and I had to go to Edgware General Hospital. I was seen by Doctor George Webster, who said after he examined me thoroughly that, there was an accumulation of fluid in my abdomen. He prescribed diuretics to get rid of the fluid, and asked me to return to the hospital to see Doctor Bevan in four weeks time.

I started to take my medication regularly, but I felt quite ill. My nose and gums started to bleed. My state of health began to deteriorate more than ever before.

After four weeks I went back to hospital to see Doctor Bevan. I was sure that he would prescribe some medicine that would help me to recover quickly.

I was told in advance that only Doctor Bevan would be able to prescribe the right medication to cure my liver, so I was desperate to see him.

At the out-patients clinic in Edgware General Hospital, Doctor Bevan examined me thoroughly. I was sitting watching him while he was looking at my file. His eyes were focused on my medical reports, then he raised his eyes slowly and looked at me as if he had an important announcement to make. "I will write to Doctor Dusheiko (now Professor Dusheiko) at the Royal Free Hospital, to examine you again to decide whether a certain medication would be a desirable treatment for your condition", he said.

When I heard these words, I became worried even more disappointed. I asked Dr Bevan instantly, what he meant by that? Doctor Bevan told me that Doctor Dusheiko is a liver specialist and a prominent consultant in liver diseases and hepatitis C, and he would consult with him to get a second opinion on a particular medication.

The question at that particular moment, was not the medication, but how I managed to reach that stage where a consultant like Doctor Bevan needed a second opinion from another specialist in another hospital. That was enough to indicate that my illness and my health condition were in a very serious state.

I had never been ill in my life, and I had never been to seek medical advice, or treatment. Now I was being seen by many doctors, going to two different hospitals, and God knows what else.

There were many questions that needed to be answered, and Doctor Bevan tried to answer as many as he could. However, I felt that there was nothing that would satisfy my curiosity, for I needed more explanations.

How could I convince myself of something I could not grasp the reasons of? There is nothing without reason or justification, that is simple logic.

I had never suffered from any illnesses or diseases. Never stayed in bed, even when I caught a bad cold, suddenly I was suffering from such a dreadful disease!

My disease must be a terrible one, otherwise why did I have to see so many doctors, and to go to see another specialist in another hospital.

I had to wait for a few weeks to see Doctor Dusheiko in the Royal Free Hospital. I phoned his secretary and I explained my condition to her. She informed Doctor Dusheiko, who was able to arrange an emergency appointment for me to see him.

The appointment was just three days before Christmas Day of 1995. That was the earliest possible appointment he could arrange.

I was working as usual, but not in my best form. In early December I attended an international conference in London, which lasted for two days. By the end of that conference, I was exhausted and feeling unwell.

I phoned my GP to arrange an appointment to see her, but I was told to go to the surgery first to have a blood test, then I would go to see her later in the week. It was obvious that she wanted to see the result of my blood test first.

I went to the surgery to have my blood test. The nurse noticed something abnormal in me. She immediately asked me whether I was going to see Doctor Pinto. I told her that I would see her in four days time. The nurse asked me to wait, till she speaks with Doctor Pinto in her consulting room.

A few minutes later, the nurse came back, asking me to go to see Doctor Pinto in her room. At the same time Doctor Pinto herself came out of her room and asked me to follow her. My wife and I followed Doctor Pinto to the consulting room. After examining me, she said that I had to go to Edgware General hospital immediately. "I will phone the hospital to tell them that you are on your way, and I will write a letter to take it with you to the doctor in the Accident and Emergency Department", she said. Then she added that she would call an ambulance to take me to the hospital. I told her that I would rather go by taxi.

Doctor Pinto asked me to wait for her in the waiting room while she was phoning the hospital. We went into the waiting room, and the receptionist came with a glass of water and asked me to drink it. I was really thirsty, but I did not ask for water, how did she know that I was thirsty? Meanwhile, Doctor Pinto came to give me the letter. The receptionist phoned for a taxi, and we went straight to the hospital.

I sat in the taxi quietly. I did not speak a word, sitting stunned by what was happening. The taxi took about ten minutes to arrive at Edgware General Hospital.

2

First Admission

As we arrived at the Accident and Emergency department at Edgware General Hospital, we went straight to the reception desk. I handed the letter in, and waited for a few minutes until a nurse came to take me to the consulting room. My wife and I, were sitting silently, waiting for the doctor to come. I was wondering, why I had to go to hospital in the first place, and why did my doctor have to send me to hospital in such a hurry? And why was I dreadfully fatigued?

All these questions remained without an answer till the doctor came. The doctor examined me, took my blood pressure and blood sample. He went away without saying very much during the whole procedure that lasted a few minutes. Everything was done with such speed that it made me worry. I was just sitting, staring, looking around, unable to talk. I was astounded by what was going on. I was expecting anything, for in a hospital anything can happen.

I waited for an hour or so till the doctor came to tell me what had happened, and what he was going to do with me.

I had never thought dreadful thoughts before, but at that particular moment I did. I was used to look on the bright side of everything, but as I was sitting, waiting, I could not afford that luxury.

This clouded scenario had barred me from seeing any brightness. All the philosophical ideas and the bright thoughts that I used to preach, had gone, and perhaps had gone for ever.

At that particular time I was confronted with the reality, the fact of life. Things that I had never contemplated, even as a nightmare, had now become reality.

Many dark thoughts came into my head as the doctor was examining me. He went and came back with a Cannula that he inserted into one of my veins. It was painful but I had to suffer in silence.

The doctor told me that I would have to stay in hospital for a few days, and I had to have blood transfusion, because the level of haemoglobin in my blood was very low.

Staying in hospital as a patient, lying in bed ill, was awful, dreadful and something that I had never experienced before.

I enquired about the possibility of going to hospital every day to receive my medication and go home as an out-patient, not as an in-patient. My request was ignored and fell on deaf ears. The reason for that was: I had to have a blood transfusion, and that could only be done as an in-patient.

I was not only worried about having to stay in hospital, but I was also worried about the idea of having a blood transfusion. I had heard and read many stories and reports about patients being given contaminated blood that caused them to contract serious diseases. I had to express my fear to my doctor, but I was assured that the blood had been screened for any contamination, and was completely clean and safe.

Two nurses came in and asked me to get on a wheelchair. I was driven in to the ward. That was difficult to accept, but I had no other alternative. I could not explain my feelings at that particular moment. I was speechless.

I had made some commitments before my doctor sent me to hospital, and I wanted to keep them. Two of these commitments were very important. The first, was an appointment to see Doctor Dusheiko at the Royal Free Hospital, in four days time, and the second was to attend an annual event in ten days time. These two appointments I did not wish to miss.

I asked the nurse to assure me that they would discharge me in three days, but I was not given that assurance. I was told that would depend on the doctors in the ward. However, when the nurse raised the matter with one of the doctors, he declined my request.

In the ward, doctors and nurses started my treatment. Every day I had in my body a pint of blood, followed by another pint of glucose. This process lasted for three days, and during those days I was feeling very uncomfortable.

I did not know how to justify what was happening. I was unable to think, my mind went blank. However much I tried, I was unable to accept what was happening to me at face value. The only thing I could think of at that time was, how could I persuade myself to except the harsh reality of life?

I was overtaken by one dream, and one hope. Who would be able to help me to recover quickly to enjoy life again?

In a couple of days I would be seen by a liver

specialist who would have the final say in this saga. I tried to imagine Doctor Dusheiko with a magic wand that could find a miracle cure that would make me recover from my illness.

The first night in hospital was a dreadful one. I was awake all night for I could not sleep at all. How could I sleep with a Cannula stuck in my arm? Furthermore, the fact that there were at least twenty-four patients sleeping in the same ward, was more than enough to keep me awake all night.

In morning, I was exceptionally glad to see the day light. Cleaners came in with their big vacuums to sweep the floor. The noise produced was mixed with the sound of patients, coming and going to and from the bathrooms, looking at me and whispering to each other.

I was like a stranger, but certainly not in paradise. Smiling and greeting other patients with one question in mind, how could I clean my teeth and wash my face with a Cannula stuck in my arm? That was beside the fact that there were too many patients and too few bathrooms.

The hospital, which has recently been closed, was an old one compared with other hospitals. However, I must admit that doctors and nurses there were doing an excellent job with their limited resources.

I lost my appetite for food, so I did not have any breakfast. All I had was, a cup of tea.

Breakfast time finished at eight thirty, and at around eleven o'clock, Doctor Bevan and Doctor Webster, together with a group of junior doctors and medical students, came to see me. I told Doctor Bevan and Doctor Webster about my two engagements. They agreed that I had to go to my appointment to see Doctor Dusheiko at the Royal Free Hospital, but they declined to make any comment on my other appointment. They told me that I could be taken directly from Edgware General Hospital to the Royal Free by an ambulance if I wanted to. I declined the offer, and I expressed my wish to go home and to go to the Royal Free Hospital in the morning by taxi.

I hated to be carried in an ambulance. I did not like to feel that I was unable to walk. I decided to go home first to have a nice warm bath, and in the morning I would go straight from home to the hospital.

During my stay in Edgware General Hospital I had about five pints of blood and five pints of glucose. I felt much better than before. That was very promising, and gave me much hope of speedy recovery. Unfortunately, that feeling and that hope did not last for long.

My wife and my daughter picked me up from the hospital and we went straight home for a nice hot bath and a nourishing meal. How much I had missed my bed, my home and every simple small thing in it.

It was the first time that I had to sleep in a hospital, and I hoped it would be the last.

After I had four days of compulsory relaxation lying ill in the hospital, and I had plenty of blood inside my blood vessels, I felt so good. I was more energetic than before.

This transformation for the better made me think that I was exhausted and after that compulsorily relaxation, I was recovered. I was determined not to allow my illness or my exhaustion to overcome me, and at that particular moment I was feeling well and it was my intention to keep it that way.

3

At The Royal Free

I slept the night at home, and in the morning I went straight to see Doctor Dusheiko in the outpatients clinic at the Royal Free Hospital. I was eager to see him. I thought of him as my saviour, the only person who could hold the key to my recovery.

I went to the reception desk and I handed in the report that was given to me by the doctor in Edgware General Hospital. It was Thursday and clinic 6 was very busy, however, I did not have to wait for a very long time.

The hospital looked well organised. It is modern, bright and more cheerful than Edgware General hospital. After nearly twenty minutes, I was called by an assistant to Doctor Dusheiko. She examined me and asked many questions that I answered with an absolute honesty. She wrote down all my personal and medical details and went to see Doctor Dusheiko in an adjacent consulting room.

A few minutes later she returned accompanied by Doctor Dusheiko who examined me again. His opinion from the start was sound and clear. I was suffering from hepatitis C and liver cirrhosis, and I needed a liver transplantation. He then added that I had to admit first to 'Hassall Ward' in the Royal Free Hospital at once to be under observation. There, I would have a complete medical assessment to see whether I was physically fit to cope with the strain of the liver transplant operation.

Immediately after I heard what he said, I started to argue with him in the belief that Doctor Bevan sent me to see him in order to seek a second opinion on a medication, not on an operation, let alone liver transplantation.

Doctor Dusheiko is an honest and kind doctor. He told me in a gentle and friendly manner that, the only suitable form of treatment that was available for me at that time was a liver transplantation. I was in need for a new liver.

I was shocked and astonished by the news. Doctor Dusheiko noticed my worry and he tried to calm me down. He tried to make me understand why liver transplantation was the best form of treatment for me. He also explained that the sooner I had a new liver, the better.

He recommended that I had to admit to Hassall Ward first for medical examinations and then they would review my health condition again. This would give them the chance to evaluate my state of health accurately.

Doctor Dusheiko sounded as if he wanted to say that I was in urgent need of a new liver, but when he noticed my facial expressions he softened his tone. Then he told me that they wanted first to examine me thoroughly, then they could decide what was necessary.

I sat silent, speechless for a few seconds. I did not know what to say or what to do. I became emotionally depressed. My brain became numb. I was unable to think or talk.

I left Doctor Dusheiko's room to go to Hassall Ward. I was walking like a robot, someone, somewhere was holding my remote control.

I felt that my hope of a speed recovery had vanished. All my dreams had been shattered. I was left with emptiness, and dark thoughts. However, I was not convinced with the idea that there was no other way to treat my illness but liver transplantation.

I was surprised to see that at the verge of the twenty first century, with its high technology in medicine and science, there is no medicine for a disease! That was impossible for me to believe. There must have been some other medication or treatment other than liver transplantation to cure chronic liver diseases. However, I had to accept what was on offer at that time, even though I was not convinced.

We were on the first floor, and we had to go to Hassall Ward on the tenth floor. I had to accept the fact that I was seriously ill.

I tried very hard to take life easy, but when I looked around, I found nothing but fear and gloom. The only bright side I could think of at the time was that I was fortunate to be in safe hands, in a hospital with a good reputation.

The liver Unit at the Royal Free Hospital is considered to be one of the best centres for liver disease, not only in the UK, but in the world. That was sufficient to give me some comfort and to be more optimistic.

In times of difficulties and uncertainties, we have to be either believers or philosophers. At that moment, I preferred to choose the former rather than the latter, and to turn my face to God, asking Him for help.

We have to create our own image of the world that suits us. A world of our own making, a world that is worth living in.

Looking on the bright side, there must be hope in life, otherwise life would not be worth living. I had to forget cynicism.

On the tenth floor, we went to the reception desk and I asked to see Doctor Pratt as Doctor Dusheiko recommended. He helped us in pre-admission formality. I signed an admission form, and we were asked to wait for a nurse to take me to my hospital bed in the Hassall Ward.

An hour later a nurse with a gentle smile Drawn upon her face came and asked me to follow her. I went with her to a small single bed room. That was in itself, a good start. Something brilliant, at least that was what I hoped for. I could wash my face and use the bathroom with absolute freedom. I was told that I would be under observation for the first three days.

It was two days before Christmas and some of the patients went home to spend the Christmas holiday with their families. The atmosphere in Hassall Ward was cheerful for the Christmas and the New Year. Everyone was smiling. Some smiling with great effort, others voluntarily, while some were smiling because they had to.

The ward was quiet, and the spirit of the Christmas was everywhere. Some nurses were busy hanging decorations around the ward and along the corridors. Illuminated Christmas trees were in every corner. It was an opportunity to make the most of the season of the good will.

Smile and the world smiles with you, be angry, and you stand alone. I was trying to smile and to be cheerful, but how when I was lying ill in bed, in a hospital, and on Christmas day. In the time that was supposed to be a happy time, but for me it was just the opposite.

Inside the room, I changed my clothes, ready for whatever was going to happen. A nurse came to take some information from me, mainly about my diet, and also to take my blood pressure and temperature. A young doctor came to take my blood sample, and a group of medical students followed. It looked as though no one wanted to miss a chance of learning something from the new patient.

In hospital, time was passing slowly, and my knowledge of how to behave as a patient was very poor indeed. I asked the nurse on duty that day to give me some ideas of what was going to happen to me, and who was going to see me. The nurse whose name is Jacqueline was very kind to me. She gave me enough information that kept me surviving the first three weeks in Hassall Ward.

On Christmas Day at lunch time, my room door was opened, A chef dressed in a kitchen uniform, with a long white hat on his head, pushed a trolley full of food into my room.

In the middle of that trolley there was a big tray with a large turkey. There were many doctors and nurses around the trolley. "Your lunch sir," the chef said with a smile.

It was not a normal hospital lunch, it was like a banquet. I never expected that kind of treatment in a NHS hospital. I expected to feel miserable and lonely during the Christmas holiday. I also expected to see that most of the medical team, from nurses to doctors to be off duty that day. However, it was to my surprise that they were all on duty.

Indeed, Hassall Ward was full of doctors that day. The tall chef with a long white hat who was serving every patient, one by one, was indeed, a very kind man.

It was a very good gesture from the hospital to let

the chef himself serve the patients on that day. The chef served my lunch, and wished me a speed recovery and good wishes for the Christmas and the new year. Later on a nurse came in with a Christmas present for me. It was a packet of handkerchiefs and a bottle of aftershave.

After the chef had gone, I discovered, and to my astonishment that, the chef was not really a chef working in the kitchen, but he was in fact Professor N. McIntyre, a prominent liver specialist in the Royal Free Hospital. He left his family in Christmas Day, and came to the hospital to serve Christmas lunch to his patients. That was splendid and considerate of him.

These small gestures helped to make my entire stay in Hassall Ward at the Royal Free Hospital more bearable.

I must admit I was a difficult patient to deal with. Asking questions and always in need for more explanations. However, I received neither the explanations, nor the answers that satisfied my curiosity.

Nurses and doctors were well aware of my worries, and they were very kind, and patient with me.

Thinking about my state of health, my life, and about what was going to happen to me, was frightening.

My thoughts were a mixture of pessimism with a little of optimism. However, I tried to conquer this feeling by some understanding of my state of health and by accepting the fact that I was ill and I was a patient lying in a hospital bed.

Life cannot and would not be all that dull. There must be something good in life to hope for.

I used to make fun of the irony of my situation, just to ease off the pain of the sad reality. It was really a funny recollection and reflection, that during my whole life, I had never been a patient in a hospital before, and all of the sudden, in a space of three days, I found myself lying in bed as a patient, not only in one hospital, but in two.

Giving my arm to a young doctor to take as much blood as she wanted for a blood test, my memory went back to the past three days. I sat, comparing the two different worlds: of Edgware General Hospital and the Royal Free Hospital. This was a good example of the past and the present, the old and the new, not only in the sense of time, but also in the sense of technology and modernity.

If I had to learn something from being in two hospitals in space of three days, it was the unfairness that exists between two different worlds, the developed and the underdeveloped. Human resources may be similar or even the same, but they are exposed to completely different circumstances.

At the Royal Free Hospital, I had to go through many series of different tests and a variety of medical examinations, some of which were very painful. I had to bear the pain in silence since I was not allowed to take any pain relief or to be under sedation. I was allowed to take only Lactulose and diuretics, and when it was necessary, I could take paracetamol. I was not allowed to take any other medication, as it would cause more damage to my liver.

Those medical examinations, which lasted for two weeks, were very tiring indeed. During this period, I was transferred from a single room, to a 4-bedded room in the same ward.

Hassall Ward is a special ward for patients with chronic liver diseases. Patients in this ward came from different social, and culture backgrounds, and also of different age groups. They all had one thing in common, they suffered from liver damage.

Some patients were addicted to either alcohol or drugs, or both, and others did not know how they contracted the disease.

A patient, aged thirty-six years, told me that he was drinking two bottles of Vodka a day, but he was determined not to drink any more. Another patient told me how drugs and alcohol had destroyed his life. He used to drink and take drugs until one day he became very ill, unable to move to go to see his doctor, or to contact a friend.

There were many sad stories like these, depressing, but interesting to learn. Doctors had to clean the blood of these patients from any traces of drugs or alcohol, before they could start their treatment for liver damage.

That was for the patients who were drinking or taking drugs, but what about patients like me who has never taken drugs, and gave up smoking and drinking for more than ten years.

It is true that I was a smoker, and I used to drink alcohol occasionally, but that was a thing of the past. I had given up all these poisons a long time ago.

However, I could understand that I was suffering from liver damage, but what I could not understand was the actual meaning and the symptoms of hepatitis C. I was unaware of such disease. I was in complete darkness about its symptoms. It was ridiculous to know so little about a virus that is spreading all over the world at an alarming nature. That was what I later discovered, but when it was too late. It is a pity that doctors and politicians did not take a drastic action to prevent these dreadful viruses from spreading.

I was determined to learn more about liver diseases. I had to read many books and medical magazines about this particular topic. However, I would not have this opportunity until I was discharged from the hospital.

I stayed in the Royal Free Hospital for nearly three weeks. During that period I was seen by nearly all the consultants specialised in liver diseases. Doctor Burroughs and Doctor Mistry were the regular consultants.

After the doctors had finished all the tests and medical assessments, I had to wait for the final result. The result that would decide my treatment. The conclusion that would shape my life to come.

4

Breaking the News

One evening, after I had my dinner, Doctor Mistry, accompanied by Linda Selves, the Transplant Assistant, came to see me. Linda handed me a booklet entitled 'Liver Transplantation, Information For Patients And Their Families.' Looking at the title was enough to put me off.

Doctor Mistry told me that the liver transplant team had completed all the medical tests and investigations, and the transplant team were satisfied to put my name on the waiting list for a liver transplantation. He also told me that my liver was damaged, and all the tests concluded that I should have a liver transplantation as soon as there was a suitable donor.

A suitable donor must have a healthy liver that matches my blood group and the size of my liver.

I tried to persuade Doctor Mistry to change his mind, and to find another method of treatment that was less risky than the transplantation. Doctor Mistry was adamant that liver transplantation was the only treatment that was suitable for me.

After more than half an hour of discussions, Doctor Mistry left me with no other alternative but to agree to the transplantation. He also left me with no doubt, that if I did not have a new liver soon, the chance of living for another year was very slim. This was the same conclusion that Doctor Dusheiko had reached.

I had to calculate all the pros and cons of the liver transplantation and above all the chance of its success.

The main argument was, if the transplantation was successful, the chance of surviving for many years was good. However, avoiding liver transplantation completely was very risky and I might not survive for even a few months. Doctor Mistry also made it absolutely clear, that the chance of a successful transplantation depends on the patient's health and age, and the younger the patient is the better.

The discussion ended with one message, transplantation was the only form of treatment available for me, and the sooner I had it, the better.

I asked Doctor Mistry to give me more time to think about it at home and after they discharged me from the hospital, but he was reluctant to agree.

Doctor Mistry left, and I asked Linda, the transplant assistant to stay for a while. I asked Linda about the operation and its success rate. I also asked her to give me her personal opinion about an alternative medicine and whether changing my life style, and following a special diet, would help me to recover from the disease.

Linda was careful not to give any medical opinion but she was a good listener, and I thought she wanted to say 'it is too late for that.'

What I wanted at that time, was to find someone who would agree with me to try something other than transplantation. Unfortunately, I could not find anyone.

Looking at Linda's facial expressions, I could easily read her thoughts, and my interpretation was that, she wanted to say that our conversation would not lead any where.

I was careful not to jump to any conclusion or to take a hasty decision that I would regret later. However, Doctor Mistry and Linda, saw my situation from a completely different perspective. They saw that I was in urgent need of a new liver, and any delay would involve taking a big risk.

Linda went to her office and I stayed by myself, thinking of what I ought to do. I had to choose between the risk of the transplantation and the risk of staying without it. It was a hard decision, and I had to take it quickly.

That night I could not sleep. I told the nurse to tell Doctor Dusheiko that I wanted to see him urgently. The next morning Doctor Dusheiko came to see me. I begged him to find any other medication or any treatment other than liver transplantation.

Doctor Dusheiko is an honest man and was frank with me. He repeated what I had been told before, that the only treatment available at that time for patients like myself, was a liver transplantation, and the sooner I had a new liver the better.

The same afternoon, a nurse told me that, I was going home, and I would come to the outpatients clinic to see Doctor Dusheiko. This meant, that they had not put my name on the waiting list for a liver transplantation. For if they had, my name would have been transferred to another waiting list, and I would be under the care of Doctor Burroughs, who normally sees liver transplant patients before and after the transplantation. That was besides the fact that, if they had, I would have been given a bleeper to facilitate hospital contact with me once they found a suitable donor.

I was very pleased to go home, but I was confused. There was no medication other than the medication I used to take before, Lactulose for constipation, and diuretics to prevent the accumulation of fluid in my abdomen. There was no medication to treat my liver damage, or even to treat the irregularity in my digestive system.

It was difficult to accept the idea of not taking any medication to treat my damaged liver. All this high technology and highly sophisticated scientific researches, and there is still no medication for liver diseases that are spreading around the world! That was hard to believe.

It was the first time that I could realise from my own experience, how inconsistent human behaviour is!

Humans have travelled into space, walked on the moon and returned to earth safely. Even as I was writing this book, drug companies have successfully discovered an anti-impotence drug, to improve the quality of life for men and another drug will be on the market, to make people lose weight and look slimmer. However, scientists have failed to find new medications to treat infected people with viruses that kill millions of people each year.

How can anyone justify the huge amounts of money that are spent every day on things that are either unnecessary or do not have priority in life. At the same time we ignore things that are essential to our existence, essential to our life!

We need to stay healthy to enjoy our living. People need a clean, and healthy environment, good hospitals and good medication, not nuclear bombs and weapons.

These philosophical ideas, or rather, these hallucinations that I thought of were a result of my frustration and despair. However, I should concentrate on matters that concern my health. What needed at that moment was a clear mind to think properly to take the right decision.

I had no other alternative, but to choose between, a new liver with the risk of rejection and infection, and taking the risk of having a slim chance of surviving for another year. It was difficult to decide.

It was helpful for me at that particular time to ask myself, whether I had any other alternative besides liver transplantation.

That question helped me a great deal in reaching the conclusion. However, I had decided that before taking any decision I had to learn more about liver diseases. I had to learn about hepatitis C as well as the risks that are involved in liver transplantation. With this in mind, I ignored every thing else. My full time occupation at that time was to concentrate on my health and to learn more about my illness.

After I was discharged from hospital, I started to visit many medical libraries. I read many medical references, borrowing as many books and medical magazines as I could. Reading day and night to find out as much information as I could about liver diseases. I became obsessed with medicine and health. I even phoned friends and relatives living abroad asking them to collect some information about the viruses that cause liver damage.

It was a challenge and a fight. A challenge to survive and a fight to defeat the disease. But how could I defeat liver cirrhosis and hepatitis C, without going through the risk of having a liver transplantation. A battle where I must admit, I was defeated.

It was shocking to learn that all research on the

causes and treatment of hepatitis C and liver cirrhoses were in their early stages at that time. Add to this, the viruses that cause liver damage, are difficult to detect.

Medical opinion says that a patient can carry the disease unknowingly for a long time and by the time it is discovered it would be too late to be treated by conventional medicine.

The liver is "an uncomplaining organ", a noble organ that is working twenty-four hours a day without stopping or complaining. But once it shows any sign of defects it may stop functioning altogether, and sudden death may happen as a result. That is the difficulty of liver diseases.

Where would all this lead me? I decided to be my own doctor, and to treat myself by myself. I had to change my old life style and to adopt a new way of life, following healthy a diet, strengthening my body's immune system, checking my teeth regularly, and taking more physical exercise.

I thought, by doing so, I might recover from my illness, leaving liver transplantation as a last resort

5

The Dentist's Chair

After I was discharged from hospital, I started to look after my health. My first stop was a visit to my dentist to find out if my teeth were in good condition. The dentist examined my teeth and gums, and started treatment. Fortunately, there was nothing wrong with my teeth a part of some scaling.

The dentist took four sessions to treat my teeth. Three of these sessions went very well, but the fourth that was supposed to be the last, went wrong.

My upper right canine started bleeding. My dentist tried to stop the bleeding but all her efforts were in vain. She had to send me to the Accident and Emergency Department at Edgware General Hospital to get a proper medical treatment to stop the bleeding.

At the Accident and Emergency department a junior doctor examined me and after she did a blood test, the result came to show that I had a 'nasty infection.' I had to admit to hospital at once and I had to stay there for two weeks.

They put me on a wheel chair again and off to the ward. Inside the ward I felt terribly unwell.

My experience in that ward was unpleasant. It was dull and depressing. It reduced my hope of a speed recovery to nil. The ward was like a hospice rather than a hospital.

I tried to be optimistic, but the general impression and the common feeling of that ward made this a heavy task indeed. The medical staff in the ward were doing their best, but there is always a limit to every thing.

I was under the care of two consultants, who prescribed a very strong antibiotic to treat the infection. They also prescribed vitamin K to stop the bleeding. The treatment went very well, and the bleeding stopped after four days, however, my treatment for the infection lasted for ten more days.

I hated that ward, I did not like to stay in it for a minute, but I had to stay till they finished my treatment. I asked the doctor either to transfer me to another ward or to discharge me from the hospital.

I was told that I had 'a nasty infection', all the hospital wards were the same and I had to stay in hospital until I made a complete recovery. What was that infection? I did not know, and I never asked.

During my stay in Edgware General Hospital, my weight increased by nearly ten kilograms. The reason for that was, an accumulation of fluid in my abdomen. Doctor Bevan came to see me in that ward and he prescribed strong diuretics.

I stayed two weeks in Edgware General Hospital then I went home. I was tired and exhausted. However, I went back immediately to my study to improve my knowledge and to learn more about liver cirrhosis and hepatitis C.

I was supposed to see Doctor Dusheiko at the Royal Free Hospital in two weeks time and I did not know what I was going to tell him. He was expecting me to tell him that I was ready for the transplantation, but in fact I was not yet ready.

When I went to see Doctor Dusheiko, he was firm, but kind. He started by asking me whether I had made up my mind and agreed to the transplantation. I told him what had happened to me since the time he had seen me in the outpatients clinic. I also raised my concern about my state of health that had started to deteriorate. I begged Doctor Dusheiko to try any medication that could help me.

Doctor Dusheiko listened to me very carefully, but he was waiting to hear my decision on the transplantation. Something that I did not dare to talk about.

He was adamant that all my pain, my suffering and also the bleeding, were just a few symptoms and signs of my liver damage. He warned me that, without having a new liver, my state of health would continue to deteriorate rapidly.

I asked Doctor Dusheiko to delay my consent on the transplantation till the next visit for I had to sort out some family affairs first.

I felt as if I wanted to ask him to give me more time to say good bye to life before I would agree to the transplantation and to the risk that was involved.

Doctor Dusheiko asked me to make an appointment to see him again in three months time. I left the clinic without knowing what to do.

I thought that three months for a clinical appointment for a patient like myself was a long time. However, I never predicted that I would be in hospital in a matter of days.

I was reading extensively to get more information on liver diseases, but the more I read the more I became confused.

Indeed I had learnt and I had known about liver

functions and liver diseases more than I needed to know. However, what was the use of all this, and what about my treatment?

A friend of mine told me that doctors in some countries treat patients with liver diseases by taking extracts from certain kinds of herbs. I thought of trying these herbs, but I changed my mind after I learnt that herbs could cause even more damage to the liver.

I was very confused. I did not know what to do. To take a decision on whether I should have a new liver was a hard one. However, the choice was limited. It was between taking the risk of the transplantation, or taking the risk of staying without any medication or treatment.

I could not decide which way I should go. It was a difficult choice to make, and a hard decision to take. Nevertheless, my state of health at that time was deteriorating rapidly and it was going from bad to worse. I was seriously ill indeed.

Looking at myself through a magnifying glass, I could not see any hope of a speedy recovery. It was as simple as that, there was no medication to treat chronic liver disease and the only available treatment was liver transplantation. Even that was not as easy as one might think, the reason was, the shortage of donors. It was a very clouded scenario, and my vision was not clear.

I gave the liver transplantation option good thought. I discussed it first, with myself, then with my wife and daughter. I had to draw a table to count all the advantages and the disadvantages. I wanted to see everything in the day light, written in black and white before taking any decision.

After many considerations I reached a conclusion: there was no other alternative but to have a liver transplantation even though it was risky.

It was the hardest and the toughest decision I had ever made. I had to agree to the liver transplantation.

I decided to give my consent to Doctor Dusheiko in my next visit when I go to see him in the outpatients clinic at the Royal Free Hospital.

Unfortunately, events turning fast. I had to admit to the Royal Free Hospital sooner than I thought. However, I did not admit into hospital voluntarily, but I had to. I did not walk to the hospital by myself, on both my feet, but I was carried in an ambulance. At least that was what I was told, because I was in a coma.

6

The Coma

I do not remember anything of what had happened to me on that particular day. I only remember that it was around two o'clock in the after noon. I was told, it was Thursday in the month of May 1996.

From that day and for the six days that followed, my clock had stopped. I was out of order. Everything became different for me. Time or no time, ill or not ill, I was in a completely different world.

The sense of time, and the feeling of pain, or existence had gone. All my senses were switched off altogether. Every day was the same for me.

I was not living my life, not for a day or two, but for six days. My batteries went flat, and I was in need of a replacement, a new lease of life, but most importantly I was in need of a new liver! However, I had to come back to life first, then anything after that would be possible.

I stayed unconscious for six days, and according

to medical terminology, I was in a coma. Well, they can call it, whatever they like, but for myself, the fact still remained. I had no feeling no senses, it was as if I was dead.

I was in another world, a world that was completely different from the one that I used to know. No news, no worry, no pain, no physical feeling, no one to talk to or even to see, nothing of that kind.

According to my wife's recollections, I became, sick, drowsy, and sleepy, then I lost consciousness.

I became stubborn, and I refused to go to hospital. She phoned a taxi to take me to hospital but I refused to go. She phoned the hospital and they sent an ambulance to carry me. I understood later on, that even the paramedics were struggling to take me with them. However, they finally succeeded to take me to the Accident and Emergency department of Edgware General Hospital.

I do not recall anything of what had happened. My memory went blank, like a computer without any software. My inner computer was broken down, and my memory had crashed. No folders, no files and no programmes, all had gone. I was plugged in to the mains, but there was no power.

I was told that the ambulance took me to Edgware General Hospital first, where I stayed for one night. Doctors and nurses there had done all they could, then they transferred me to the Royal Free Hospital.

At the Royal Free Hospital doctors and nurses had done all their best to bring me back to life. However, I did not remember anything at all. I only remember that particular moment when I was trying to regain consciousness and come back to this world.

I was struggling hard till I became slightly conscious, then I started to wake up slowly from a dreadful and deadly sleep.

It was dark, and I did not know where I was.

I touched my face with my fingers. A mask was covering my mouth and my nose. I tried to take the mask off my mouth, but immediately I was surrounded by a crowed of people, shouting here and there. "Do not remove this" , and "do not touch that". I did not understand what all the fuss was about. I did not know what they wanted from me.

The light was switched on and I could see some people in blues and some in whites. A female voice came closer to my ears, asking me, whether I knew where I was.

I looked at her and a beautiful smile was drawn on her face, then she repeated again the same question in a very soft voice. I answered her in a very faint voice: 'No I do not,'

'You are in the Royal free hospital.'

'But who brought me here?'

'You were very ill.'

'I want to get out of bed'

'You cannot move, please stay in bed and do not try to remove the oxygen mask or the tube from your mouth and nose.'

'But I want to get out of bed'

'In the morning'

'You just go to sleep now, and in the morning you would be able to get out of bed.'

The lights were switched off and the room became dark again. The crowed had gone and I was left alone.

I could not wait till the morning. I was eager to get up and to get out of bed immediately. I tried to get out of bed, but I failed, then I tried again many times , but I failed every time. I had neither the energy nor the power that could give me the strength to be able to get up.

I kept trying. Finally I succeeded in getting out of bed. But when I tried to stand on both my feet, I fell down on the floor unable to move. The nurses came running, they carried me in such hurry and put me back to bed.

I did not know whether they gave me something to make me sleep or not, but I did not feel anything till the morning.

In the morning I opened my eyes, to found two student nurses, standing by my bed trying to wake me up. When I became slightly conscious, they washed my face and started to feed me.

These two student nurses were the first human faces that I could recognise in my second chance of life. They were the most beautiful creatures I have ever seen. Unfortunately, I do not know where they are working now.

How much I missed the pleasure, the joy and the beauty of life when I was in a coma. I did not see anyone, there was no beauty at all. It was all doom and gloom. After all Life is worth living.

It is amazing that we never appreciate many things in life until we lose it. That is people's attitude to life. It is sad but true.

I was transferred to a 4-bedded room, where I was seen by many doctors. My wife and my daughter came to see me and to their surprise they found me sitting in bed. It was a great moment to see my wife and my daughter again. It was a wonderful reunion.

I started to inquire about what had happened to me. It was unbelievable to hear about things that I had never anticipated. It was like a science fiction that I had never visualised.

However, for some reason I did not like to know all the details of what had happened. I had returned to life safely, and that was the most important part of the drama. It was the beginning of a new chapter in my life, and I must enjoy the gift of this new lease of life.

It is wonderful to have another chance to live life again. It is marvellous to look at things in different perspectives and to appreciate things that I had always taken for granted.

It was a miracle to be alive again. It proves without doubt that our existence in life has a purpose and a reason and only God knows the secret of it.

I had to resume my life again. For what purpose, only God knows! Some call it a mystery, but I call it, 'the Will Of God.'

Going back to what had happened to me, and thinking of people who argue about legalising euthanasia, I can only say, that they would be better to think again.

I was about to reach the end of the tunnel many times, and every time I lost hope in life, I found that another tunnel had been opened for me to renew my hope again.

I cannot provide any explanation for how this had happened to me other than it is 'the Will Of God,' and I will never intervene in His Will.

In the ward, doctors and nurses began their medical examinations and assessments to evaluate my state of health. There was no more time to waste.

The underlying question was, would I agree to have a new liver? The answer to this question required one word only, it was either yes or no.

I had to agree to have a new liver, and to accept the risk that was involved in the transplantation. I was quite happy to say YES.

It was amazing, that my worry of the risk of rejection and infection that I used to fear before the coma, had been completely forgotten. It was a thing of the past.

My main concern at that time was, how to look after my health and how to stop any further decline in my general condition. Doing that would help me in coping with the physical strain of the transplantation.

Before I was discharged from the hospital they

gave me a bleeper, which confirmed that I was on the waiting list for a liver transplantation. I went home, thinking that I should not take any risks that may jeopardise the transplantation.

As a matter of fact, the coma had changed my way of thinking. Why should I worry about the risks that are involved in transplantation? It did not matter any more.

I was saved many times. Someone, somewhere, wanted me to stay alive. I survived the coma, so I would also survive the transplantation.

The waiting period was the most frustrating and stressful time. I was not sure for how long I would be waiting for the transplantation. I was told that the average waiting time was between six to eight weeks. But nothing was certain. In my case, it took the hospital more than eight months to find a suitable donor.

I knew it would be a long process and a long wait, however, I had no other alternative but to wait and be patient.

7

The Transplantation

The waiting period was the most difficult time I had ever faced. I did not know when I would be called for the transplant operation. It was certainly outside my control as well as anyone else's control.

I was told that there is no numerical order of priority on the waiting list. Each patient is assessed individually according to their blood group and weight and the most suitable patient is chosen for the donor liver.

This meant that I would have to wait for any length of time. No suitable donor, no liver transplantation, it was as simple as that. However, it is sad to think that someone has to die for someone else to live.

I was also told that one of the transplant assistants would phone me when there was a suitable donor liver. This call is usually made at any time of day or night.

Not Knowing what the next hour would bring,

made me worry all the time. It was dreadful not even being able to organise my daily life. I was living minute by minute, taking whatever came.

The hospital gave me a booklet containing information on liver transplantation. It was specially produced to give information on liver transplant operations for patients and their families to read. In my opinion it is a very useful booklet, but I was puzzled by what I had read about the Waiting Period. The information are true, and correct, but it is difficult to accept. It tells patients to be ready at any time to be called, and to be prepared accordingly.

The average waiting time was between six and eight weeks, however, that was not certain, for I had to wait for more than eight months. It is true that some patients waited for only two or three months, but that is not always the case.

Nevertheless, the most worrying thing at that time was the rapid deterioration of my health. Night time was a nightmare, and day time was boring. Loss of my appetite became permanent. Life became dull, tiresome and without reason. Lack of concentration made my life even worse. Reading a book or a newspaper, or even watching a television programme without being able to concentrate, was terrible for me.

The liver transplant team were aware of all these symptoms. They knew that the waiting period could be stressful and frustrating, but it was outside their control. No one was able to do any thing.

During the waiting period, I used to go to see Doctor Burroughs every two weeks at the outpatients clinic and I had to have blood tests on a regular basis. Doctors and transplant assistants were aware of my state of health, but nothing could be done or even changed.

I was only allowed to take diuretics, to prevent the retention of fluid in my abdomen. Any other medication would harm my liver even more.

I was under a strict 'no salt diet' and I was allowed to have only 1000 ml of fluid to drink a day.

Food without salt tasted awful, but I had to eat it. I was told that I had to eat as much as I could in order to build up my tissues, and to be able to bear the physical strain that is required for any major operation such as transplantation. It was a very difficult formula, that was hard to solve. I had no appetite, but I had to eat.

I knew that many patients died while they were waiting for a suitable donor. The waiting period was a very crucial period for me and for my family. I did not know what the future would hold for all of us.

Despite everything, the waiting period made me forget the risks that were involved with the liver transplantation. All I wanted at that stage was to be called into hospital either for the transplantation, or for any form of medical treatment. Staying at home doing nothing but watching my health deteriorating rapidly and waiting for the worst to happen, was awful.

I could not bear to stay like that any longer, but nothing could be done. My patience was running out. The question that occupied my mind at that stage was, who could help me to get out of the turmoil that I was in!

Three months passed and my name was still on the waiting list. One evening, just after eleven o'clock, my telephone rang. It was Amanda the transplant assistant. She asked me to go to hospital for the operation, but she cautioned me that I might not have the liver transplantation done. However, there was a slim chance that it may be done.

It is hospital practice, that when a suitable donor is found, the transplant assistant has to phone two patients to ask them to go to hospital to be prepared for the transplantation. They normally call the first and the second on the waiting list, unless there is another patient in a critical state of health. If the first patient on the list is found to be unfit for the operation, then the second patient will be ready to have the donor's liver instead. The practice is to insure that the donor's liver is not to be wasted.

I was the second on the waiting list, so I went to hospital as I was told. I arrived there by midnight. Doctors prepared me for the operation, and I was ready. By six o'clock in the morning I was told that the donor's liver went to the first patient on the waiting list.

I had to return home disappointed, but being called into hospital for the operation, was in itself promising. It made me feel that I was not forgotten, and there was still hope.

However, I started to lose hope again. Six months had passed since my name was put on the waiting list, and my state of health was deteriorating rapidly.

I expressed my concerns to my doctor, who told me again that nothing could be done.

By the end of the sixth month, the hospital called me again at about midnight. At that time I was the first on the waiting list. I went to hospital and again doctors and nurses prepared me for the operation. However, by four o'clock in the morning a doctor informed me that the hospital received information that the donor's liver was fatty. The donor's liver was not suitable for the transplantation.

Once again, I was disappointed when I heard the news. By eight o'clock in the morning I left the hospital and went home feeling miserable.

I was looking desperately for someone who could offer me any help a part from some vague words to calm my fears or to cheer me up. But I could not find anyone.

My state of health was declining, and I was very worried that by the time the hospital could find me a suitable donor, it would be too late. However, I had no other choice but to wait patiently, praying to God, and hoping for the best.

I am a firm believer in fate. Everything has its own time, and the time for the transplantation had not come yet.

I knew I would not gain anything from worrying, on the contrary it would make matters worse. I also knew that I would be better off if I could afford the luxury of being patient, hopeful and optimistic. However, I tried to be cheerful and hopeful, but sometimes pessimism defeated the object.

Chatting over the phone was a sort of outlet, and sometimes it helped in changing my mood. Going to hospital for pre-transplantation check-ups, and mixing with other patients who shared the same suffering, helped me a great deal at that crucial time, the waiting period.

Eight months and half had passed and nothing happened. One Thursday I went as usual to the out-patients clinic for the regular check-up. On that day, I was on the verge of losing hope completely. All my strength had failed me. I met a friend whom I had not seen for a long time. I told him my story with the liver disease, and how much I suffered from it. We ended the conversation by asking him to pray for me.

I went home, walking in absolute silence. I did not want to talk, and I did not want even to hear anyone talking. My wife tried hard to engage me in talking to her, but I kept quiet, speechless. I felt as if I was in a vacuum, not living in the real world. I kept myself to myself for the whole day.

In the evening I went to bed trying to sleep, but as usual, I could not. I stayed in bed awake, and at eleven o'clock the telephone rang. The transplant assistant was on the other end, asking me to go to hospital for the transplantation.

I knew I must go, and I knew in advance that I would come back home in the morning, just as usual. It happened twice before, why could not happen this time as well.

I was certain that this call would be like the previous calls, nevertheless, I had to go anyway.

As usual I took my personal things in a bag, and before I left home to go to hospital with my wife, I told my daughter not to worry about anything for I would be back in the morning.

I went as usual to Gloucester Ward. Doctors and nurses started to prepare me for the operation. I was sure that they were wasting their time and their efforts. However, they had to do their duty since it was difficult for anyone to predict anything at that stage.

I was hoping that, this time they would operate on me. My blood test was taken, and they sent me for an X-ray, again as usual. My wife was sitting beside me talking, and suddenly I dozed off. I did not feel myself, for I was in a deep sleep.

It is the hospital's general practice, that amongst the preparation for the transplantation, doctors have to give some medication to make the patient feel drowsy and sleepy. That was what happened with me in case they operated on me.

At some point I was slightly unconscious, but I was aware of some of the things that were around me.

I remember seeing someone holding my hand, she was the transplant assistant. After that I did not feel, hear or see anything.

When I opened my eyes again, it was dark, and I did not know where I was. A nurse was sitting close to me, and I understood later, that I was in the Intensive Care Unit.

I was feeling thirsty, and I asked for a glass of

water, but I remember the nurse declined my request. Despite her gentle kindness, she was very strict. She wet my lips with a small piece of sponge soaked in water, but that did not stop me from feeling thirsty.

I stayed two days in the intensive care unit, then they transferred me to Hassall Ward. I was in a state of hallucination and confusion, sometimes I had nightmares, and sometimes I had happy dreams.

I felt as if I was in full control of myself, but in fact, I was not. It was all hallucination and confusion. I was very moody indeed. There were some faces that I did not like to see at all. Like and dislike were matters of no reason or justification.

I was aware of what was going on around me but unable to speak. I was confused, unconscious most of the time. Nurses at Hassall ward were very kind and patient but I could not help being nonsensical sometimes.

The first two weeks after the transplantation were very hectic indeed. Doctors and nurses were monitoring every stage and I had to take big doses of different kinds of medication every day.

It was unbelievable to think that the liver transplant operation was over, and I had a new liver. Above all I was saved.

It is good to be alive, although I was feeling unwell at the time. I was under the constant care of Doctor Burroughs, Mr. Rolles, and Doctor Mistry together with the rest of the transplant team.

I was surprised to see Doctor George Webster in Hassall Ward among the transplant team. I saw him for the first time when I was a patient in the Edgware General Hospital. He and his consultant Doctor Bevan, at that time, transferred me to the Royal Free hospital.

I was very pleased to see him again. I understood that he is working at the Royal Free Hospital after Edgware General Hospital was closed.

By the middle of the second week after the operation, I started to remember some poems of famous Arab and British poets. For an unexplained reason, I started to recite some of these poems to my wife and my daughter. I did not know whether that was a sign of hallucination and confusion, or a sign of regaining my mental as well as my physical health. However, just remembering those poems in such circumstances made me happy. It gave me a good reason to be confident and optimistic.

I stayed in hospital for four weeks. During that time, transplant assistants, nursing staff, physiotherapists and dieticians, gave me all the support, and help that I needed to cope with my new life at home.

Going home was the biggest step on the way to my recovery. I had to be very careful for at least the first six months. I had to monitor carefully my daily life and spot any sign of infection or rejection.

My medications included among others, high doses of immunosuppressive to bring any sign of rejection under control. It also has some undesirable side effects. It suppresses my immune system to prevent it from rejecting the new liver, but at the same time it decreases its ability to fight infections.

I had to take a great care especially in the first six months, and till my immune system regained some of its resistance to fight some infections, unfortunately, not all.

I was happy to go back home after a very hectic time in hospital. However, I was very worried and afraid of what might happen. My family and my friends made my life at home quite pleasant and comfortable. They made me forget, some of the time, that I have a foreign organ inside my body.

Immediately after I was discharged from the hospital, I felt sever back pain. I phoned the transplant assistant at the Royal Free hospital and I told her about my back pain. She asked me to come to the hospital immediately.

Doctors examined me, and I had to admit to Hassall Ward for two weeks. I developed Osteoporosis, a disease that makes bones brittle. It was a side effect of one of the medications called prednisolone.

This medication is a steroid, that I had to take in a large doses after the transplantation. It is an anti-rejection medication that also blocks some of the cells that trigger a rejection response.

This medication is a very strong one, however, it was necessary to take it. Doctor Burroughs and Doctor Mistry decided to take me off this medicine and to replace it with new a medication.

The side effects of the new medication were bearable, but still undesirable. Nevertheless, there was no other alternative.

It was difficult to think of any medication that has no side effects at all. However, I was happy with the side effects of the new medication, since that would prevent my body from rejecting my new liver. That was the most important element of any transplantation.

8

One Year After

The first year after any major surgical operation is indeed a very important one. In my case its importance lay in the way that my new liver would function in its new environment, inside my body.

The year that followed my liver transplantation, was the year that the actual assessment for any signs of progress or improvement in my health had to be made.

I expected to notice, a major change in my general health after a month or two of my transplantation.

I thought that during the first few months that followed my operation, I would notice my physique going back to its normal condition, as if nothing had happened. That was, of course, wishful thinking, or perhaps I was just overoptimistic.

However, it was unrealistic to think or even to assume that after a long period of illness, and after a liver transplantation that my health would go back to its normal healthy state.

Just imagine waking up and finding a complete stranger lying beside you in bed. That was exactly what I had imagined. A new organ, had all of the sudden found itself lying beside other strange organs in my body.

My body and my other native organs, had discovered a new liver, an intruder, an outsider trying to invade their privacy in their own territory.

In my transplantation, a new liver replaced my old damaged one. This foreign organ, even though it is good and well behaved, would be rejected if either my body or my new liver had not learnt or trained themselves to live with each other, peacefully and in complete harmony.

My new liver must find some sort of accommodation, if not complete harmonisation with my other organs. It had to get used to the new way of life, inside my body. Any rejection from any side, would put my life in a great danger.

That was why I had to take huge doses of medications regularly to tame my other organs, as well as my body to treat the newcomer in a more decent way, and not to reject each other. However, that was of course at a price.

I had to take anti-rejection (immunosuppressive) medications that helped to stop my body's immune system from attacking and rejecting the newly transplanted liver.

This medication like any other medication had beneficial effects, beside the undesirable side effects, and if I have to accept one I should have to accept the other.

I have to get used to the side effects of the anti-rejection drugs (immunosuppressive medications) or at least to learn how to live with it.

That meant, my life and my state of health would

never be the same again, however, I felt much better after the transplantation.

The main objective of the liver transplant operation, as a medical treatment is, "to improve the quality of life". My state of health has improved and I became much better than before the operation, but certainly not as I had been before my illness.

I thought that I would be able to resume my normal life once I had a new liver, but unfortunately that was not the case.

It is just impossible for anyone with an organ transplanted in their body to lead a healthy normal life style as if nothing had happened. I certainly could not conceive that. Even if I became more energetic than before, the facts still remained, I could not forget that I had a liver transplantation. A foreign body that is fighting hard to accommodate itself with the other native organs inside my body.

Immediately after the operation I learned to moderate my high expectations, and to be more realistic. I should not expect to enjoy completely normal health, but I should learn how to make do with what is left. I also had to adapt myself to the best way in dealing with the side effects of the anti-rejection medication.

I am regaining my strength slowly but surly, and I am also regaining resistance to some infections. However, any sign of rejection or infection or even a rise in temperature was enough to make me worry.

My doctors have assured me day in and day out, that my new liver is functioning very well, as a normal liver. They also asked me to be patient in dealing with the side effects of the medication which were sometimes unpleasant.

However, during the first year after the transplantation, I developed a hernia. I was advised by my doctor to have the hernia repaired one year after my transplantation.

A year later, I had to go to hospital for an annual check-up. This is done routinely, annually to all liver transplant patients. A routine liver biopsy was also to be performed after the first year to check the condition of the new liver. The result of the annual check-up was good, and my new liver is working normally.

Three months later, and I had to go into hospital for a hernia repair. My physician consultant transferred me to Mr. Rolles, the consultant surgeon, who had performed my liver transplant operation.

Mr. Rolles examined me and he agreed to go on with the hernia repair. The operation was performed and it was successful.

Hernia repair was the first real test, proved without doubt that my new liver was functioning well. However, sometimes it is difficult to control events. On the contrary events can control us most of the time. The biochemical changes, and the stress that follows any major operation, make it difficult to be optimistic all the time.

I could not pretend that I was in full control of my health after the transplantation and while I still taking the anti-rejection medication. I believe that once the human function curve starts to fall, it is difficult to make it rise again. But it is always good to try to slow it down and not let it fall fast.

Adapting a positive attitude in life can help in bringing health and happiness. Excessive burden and pressure, can bring exhaustion that reduces the ability of the body to fight illness and disease. Rightly or wrongly, that is what I believe.

In my case I am convinced that I have another chance to resume living my life again, however, not from the beginning. I am also aware that I was given a 'second hand' spare part to replace the one that was damaged.

This way of thinking helped me a great deal to take life easy, and to accept certain conditions, and to follow a certain routine in my life. I also have to accept happily that anything might happen to me. Life is so precious, and I must enjoy the rest of it to the full.

Liver transplantation is a major and risky operation, but it is the only available treatment at present to cure chronic liver diseases. For this reason I am determined to make it a success story. I must prove with evidence that one can live happily with a foreign organ.

However, I had to go to the operating theatre again for the third time in the space of sixteen months. This time was to remove an obstruction in my bile duct. The symptoms were, feeling unwell and itching all over my body, with some swelling around my abdomen.

I went to see Doctor Burroughs in the out-patients clinic without any prior appointment. I was referred to one of his assistants, Doctor James O'Brain.

I found Doctor James, friendly and he has a good sense of humour that helped to facilitate our communication and understanding, and subsequently, I trusted his opinion. He prescribed a medication and told me that he would inform Doctor Burroughs about my condition.

As I gathered, all doctors who see transplant patients in the out-patients clinic, work as a team. They review each patient's case in their meetings at the end of each working day with Doctor Burroughs, the consultant physician and Mr. Rolles the consultant surgeon.

The medication that I was given to treat itching did not work well, on the contrary the itching had increased. I had to go to see my doctor again. My doctor sent me to the ultrasound scan department to have a clear picture of my liver to assess the blood flow to and from my liver.

I went to the ultrasound department to have my liver scanned. The doctor there spotted an obstruction in my bile duct. He wrote his report, and I went immediately to see Doctor Burroughs in Hassall ward. There I met with Doctor O'Brain who after reading the ultrasound report, told me that I had to admit to the hospital. I had to stay one night for an 'ERCP.' It was a keyhole surgery to look into my bile duct and if necessary to insert a piece of plastic tube into it. The day of the admission was set, and it was in a weeks time.

The following day, was Friday, the 5th June 1998. It was the day that the Liver Transplant Unit at the Royal Free Hospital celebrated its first 500 liver transplant operations. I attended the reception that marked this occasion. Unfortunately, I could not attend the second celebration that was held in October the same year to mark the 10th anniversary of the first liver transplantation at the Royal Free Hospital.

The first celebration was well attended and successful. It was attended by the Health Secretary Mr. Frank Dobson and professor G. Dusheiko, Doctor A. K. Burroughs, Mr. K. Rolles and Doctor D. Patch, and the rest of the liver transplant team. Many transplant patients also attended.

I had the opportunity on that day to see many liver transplant patients, some of them had the transplantation twice. All of them were looking fit and well.

I was really surprised to see that their health had improved. Their features have changed to the degree that it was hard to recognise each other. They had gained weight, and their faces look healthier than before.

Four days later and I had to admit to hospital for the ERCP. I went to hospital at 8 o'clock in the morning, and by 10 o'clock the ERCP was done. I slept the night in hospital and in the morning I went home, feeling quite well.

Two weeks later I had a fever, my temperature was high and I had to phone Geraldine the liver transplant assistant to tell her about the development. She asked me to go to hospital immediately.

I went to the Accident and Emergency Department first, then I was transferred to Hassall Ward. I stayed there for a week, under observation.

My treatment included large doses of antibiotics. I was told that there was a narrowing in my bile duct and I had to be seen by Mr. Rolles for a medical examination prior to a surgical operation in my bile duct.

Mr. Rolles sent me a letter fixing the date of the operation. I knew that bile duct reconstruction, as they call it in medical terms, is a big operation and is not an easy one.

On the eve of the operation I went to hospital, and the next morning Mr. Rolles performed the operation. It lasted four and half hours, and it was done by Mr. Rolles himself.

Mr. Rolles and his team came to see me after the operation and he told me that the operation was big and not as he had expected. However, a stint must be inserted in my bile duct in three weeks time.

I was discharged from the hospital after a week, however, I had to return to have the stint inserted in my bile duct. Doctor Dooley who is another consultant in the transplant team, performed it successfully. Under anaesthetic he inserted a small fine tube made of plastic, through my throat and into my bile duct.

This surgery did not include any scars or openings, but it was a delicate one. It complemented the bile duct reconstruction. I stayed in hospital for a week then I went home.

All these operations would never have been

thought of let alone carried out, if I did not have a new liver.

My new liver has tolerated all these surgical operations and that was another convincing proof that my liver is working well. However, I still believe that there is nothing better than our natural organs, the ones that I was born with. But when there is no other alternative one can make do with any thing since it will save lives. Luckily, the alternative is working very well for me.

Sometimes I wonder why drug companies with their huge funds and research centres are unable to discover, up till now, any medication to treat chronic liver diseases. There are millions of people around the world who are suffering from these terrible liver diseases, and there are thousands of people who die every day from the lack of treatment.

It is an awful thing for anyone to think that someone has to die in order to treat someone else. I did not like it and I never will, but nothing can be done since it is the only available treatment!

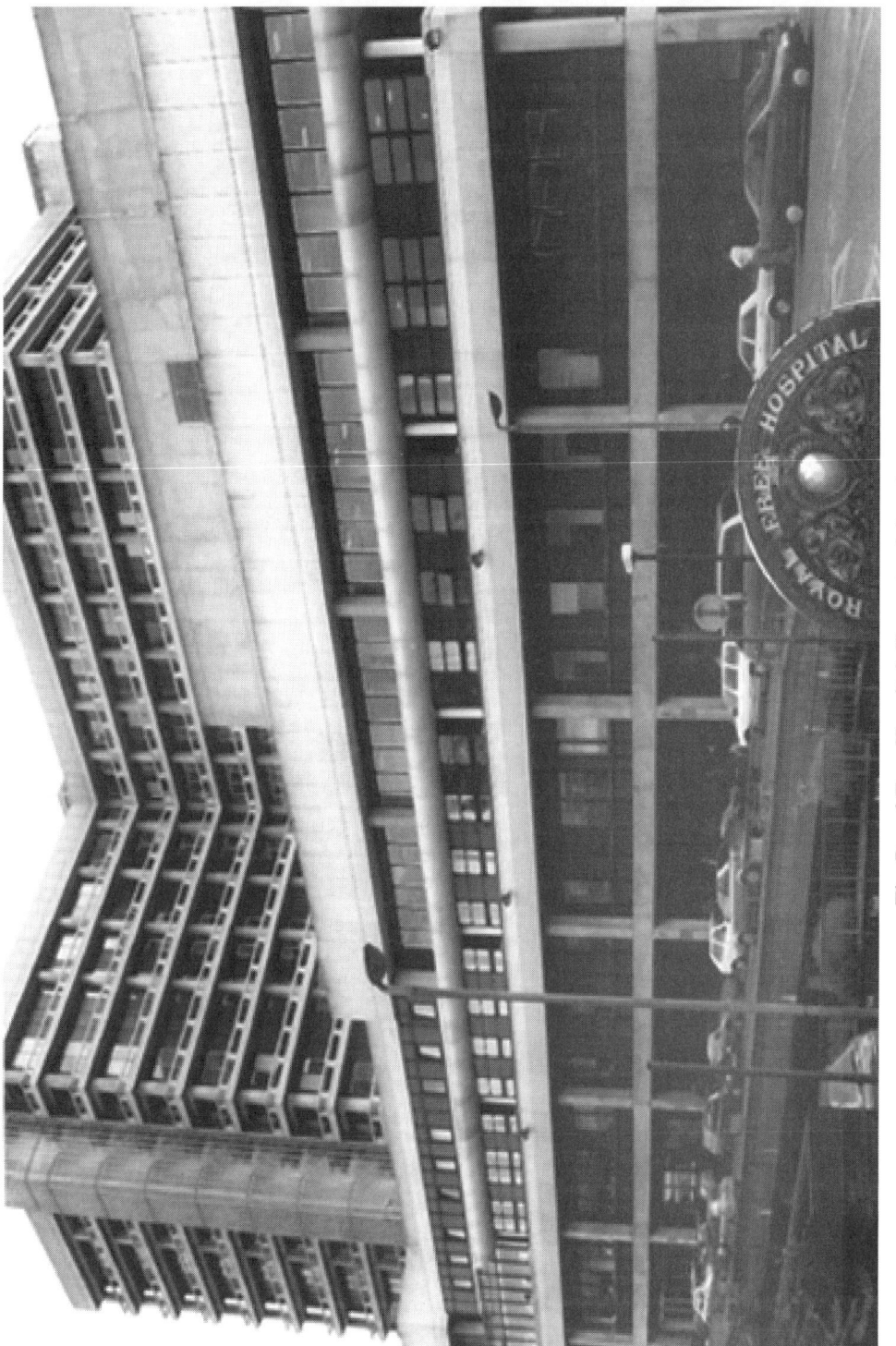

The Royal Free Hospital, Hampstead, London

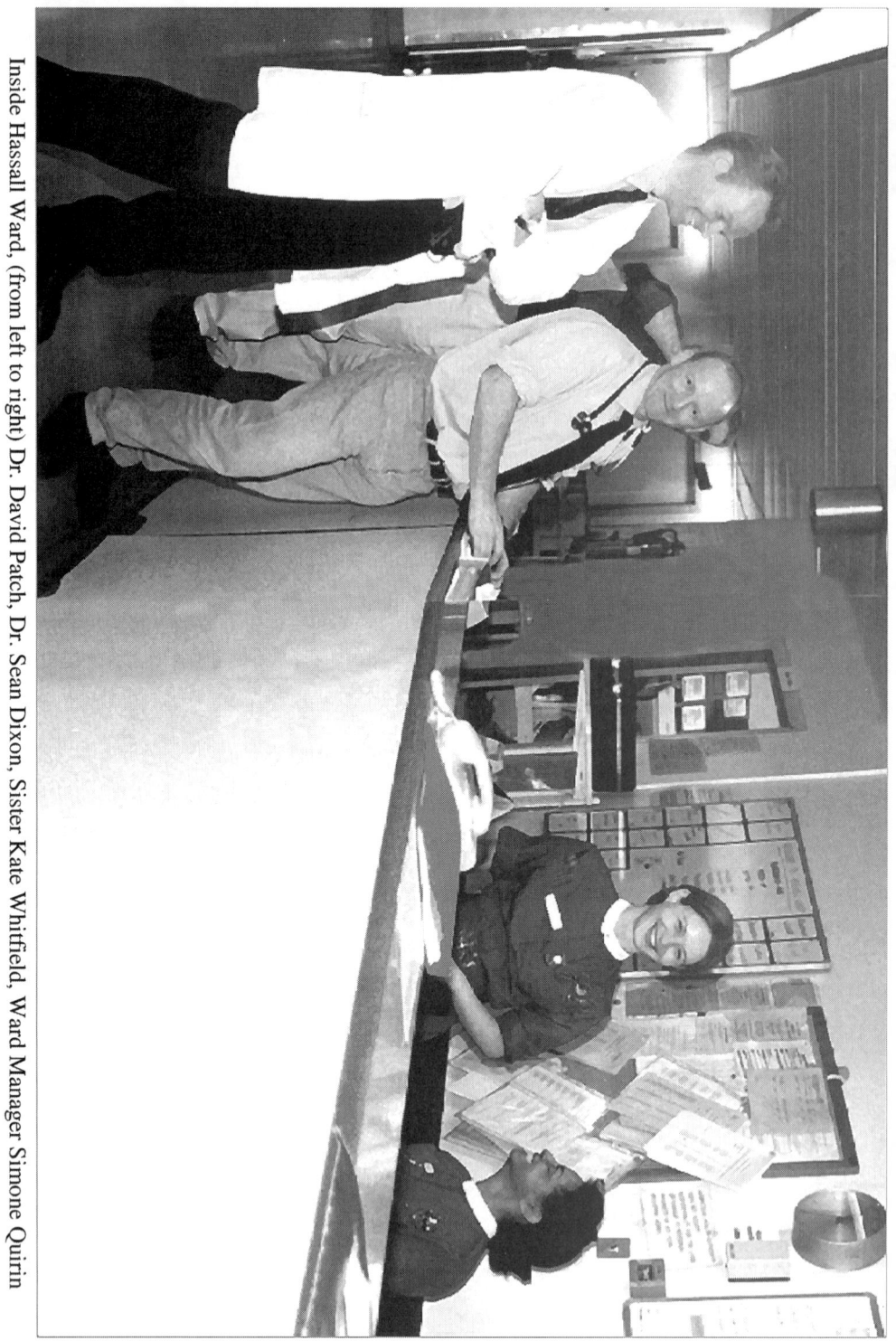

Inside Hassall Ward, (from left to right) Dr. David Patch, Dr. Sean Dixon, Sister Kate Whitfield, Ward Manager Simone Quirin

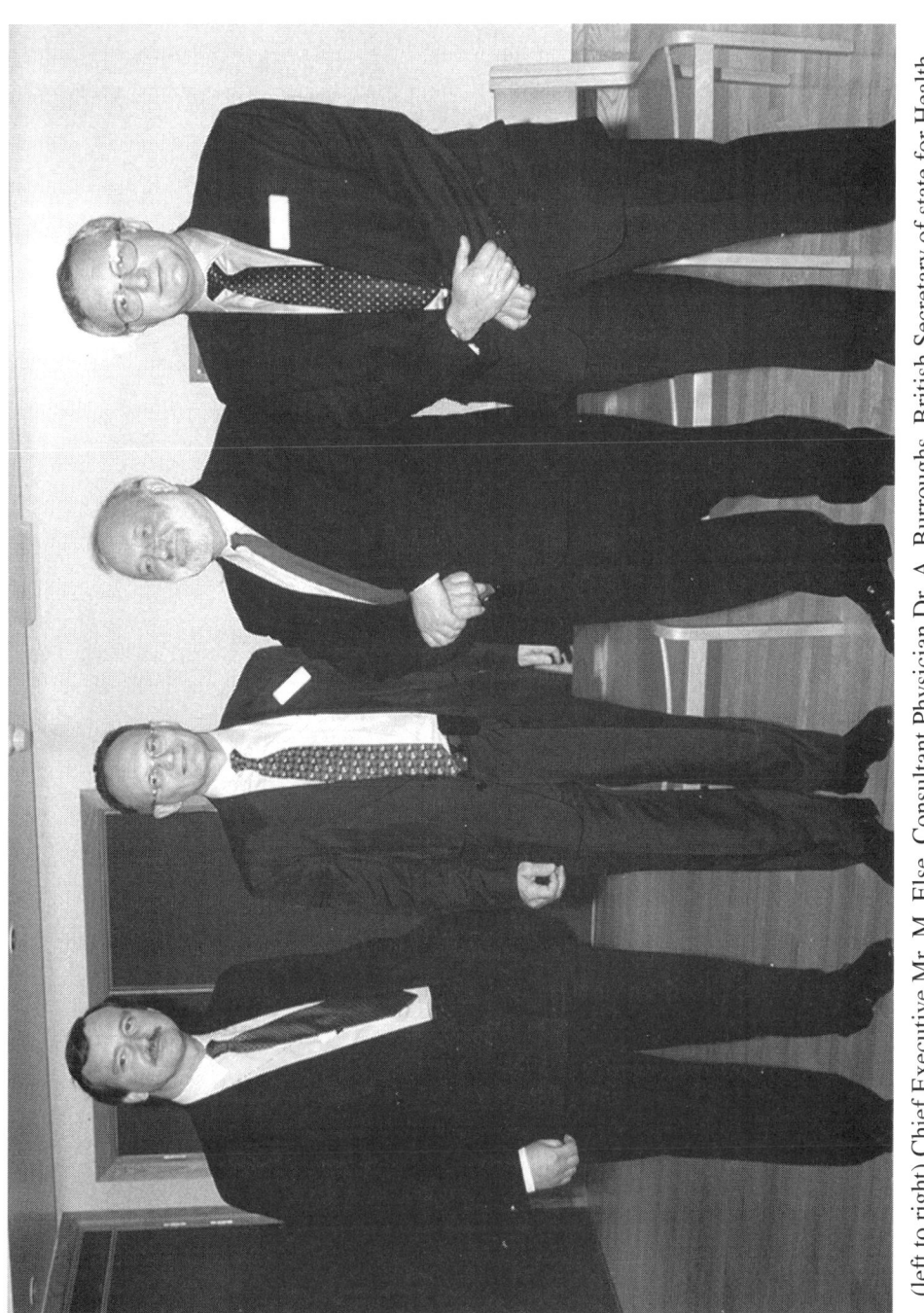

(left to right) Chief Executive Mr. M. Else, Consultant Physician Dr. A. Burroughs, British Secretary of state for Health Mr. Frank Dobson MP, Consultant Surgeon Mr. K. Rolles.

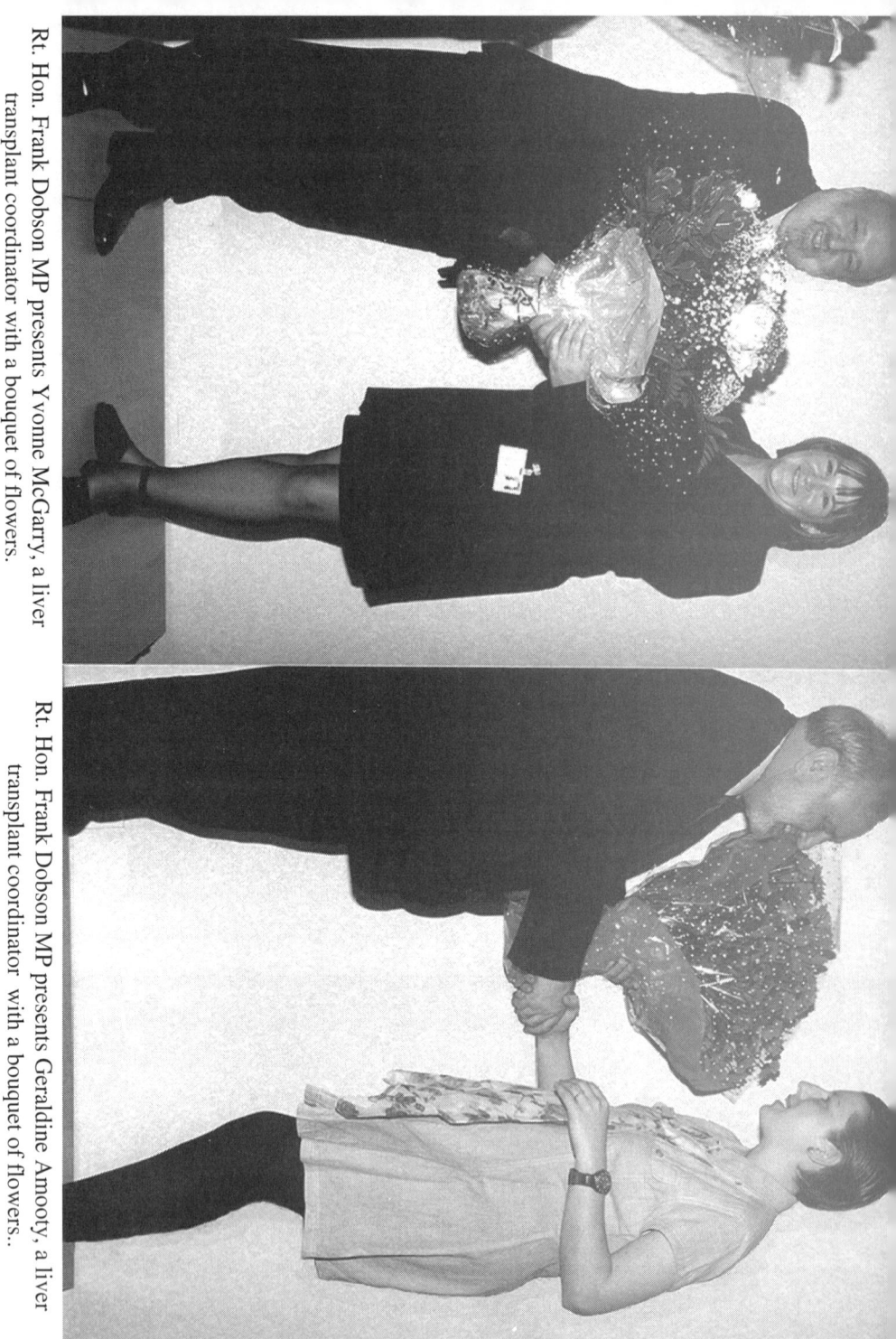

Rt. Hon. Frank Dobson MP presents Yvonne McGarry, a liver transplant coordinator with a bouquet of flowers.

Rt. Hon. Frank Dobson MP presents Geraldine Amooty, a liver transplant coordinator with a bouquet of flowers..

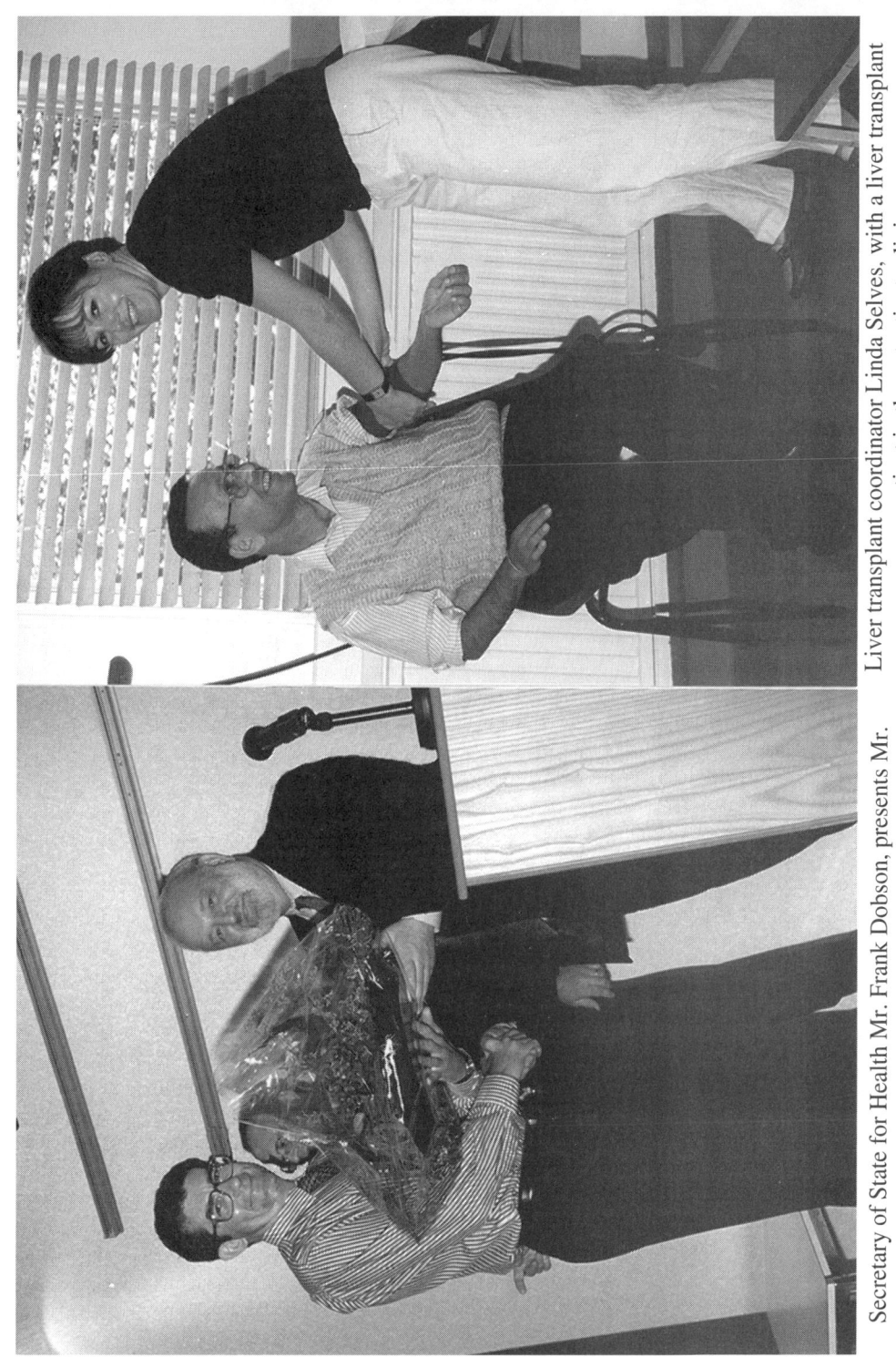

Secretary of State for Health Mr. Frank Dobson, presents Mr. Larry Davies Business manager with a bouquet of flowers.

Liver transplant coordinator Linda Selves, with a liver transplant patient in the outpatients clinic.

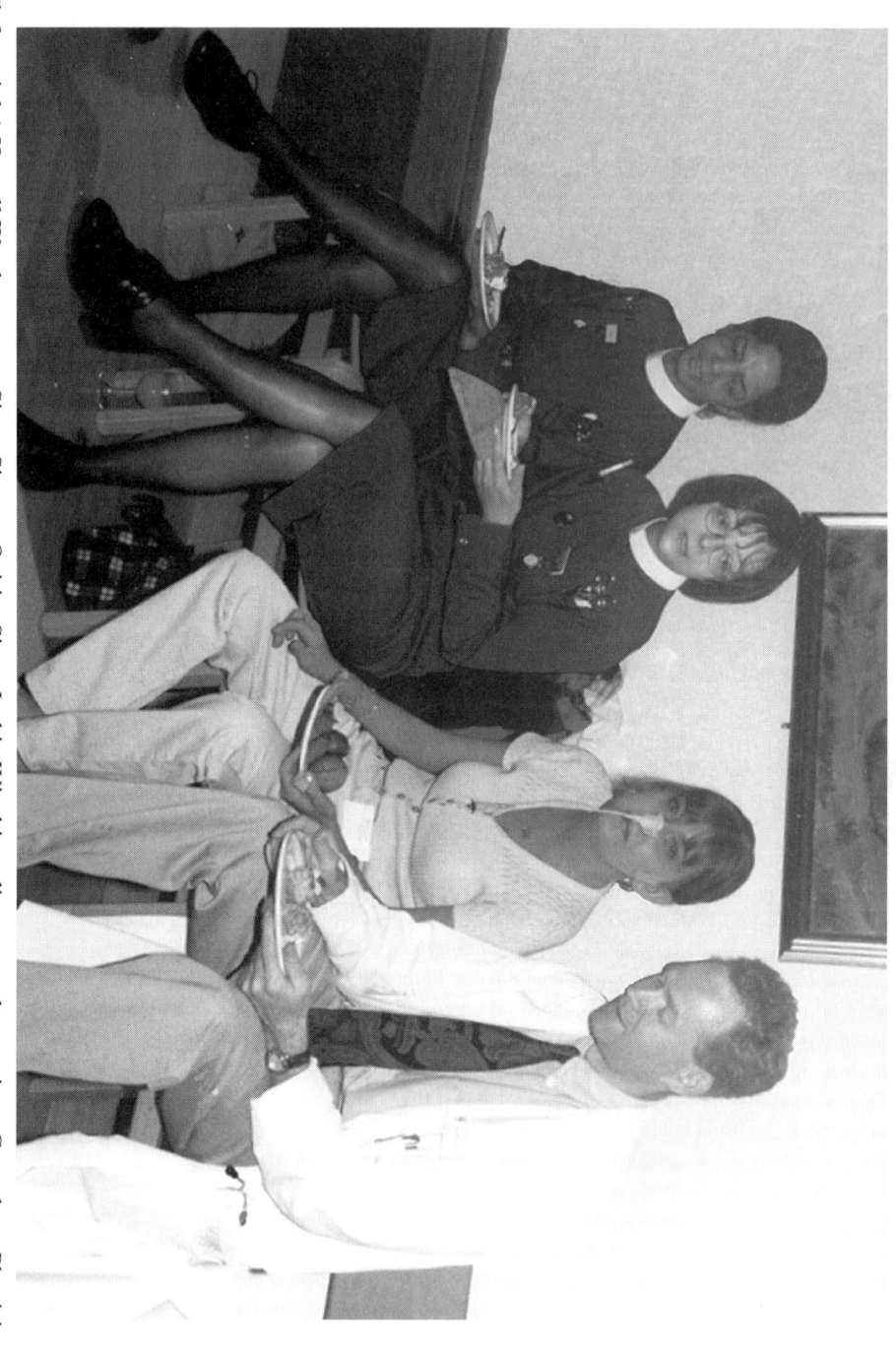

(left to right) Hassall Ward manager, Sister Simone Quirin, Sister Jackie Winship, a liver transplant patient, Consultant Physician Dr. David Patch at celebration of 500 liver transplants at the Royal Free Hospital.

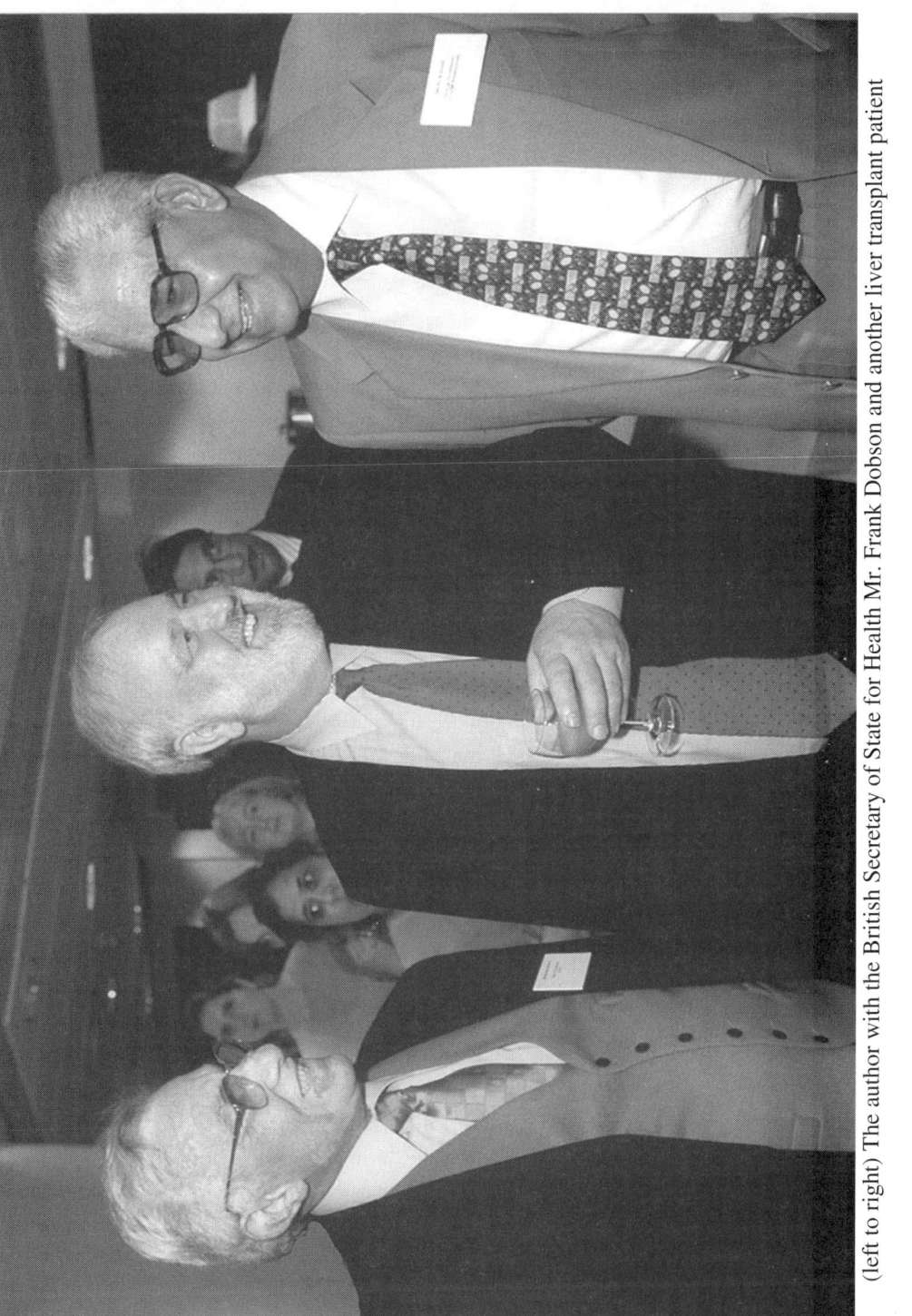

(left to right) The author with the British Secretary of State for Health Mr. Frank Dobson and another liver transplant patient

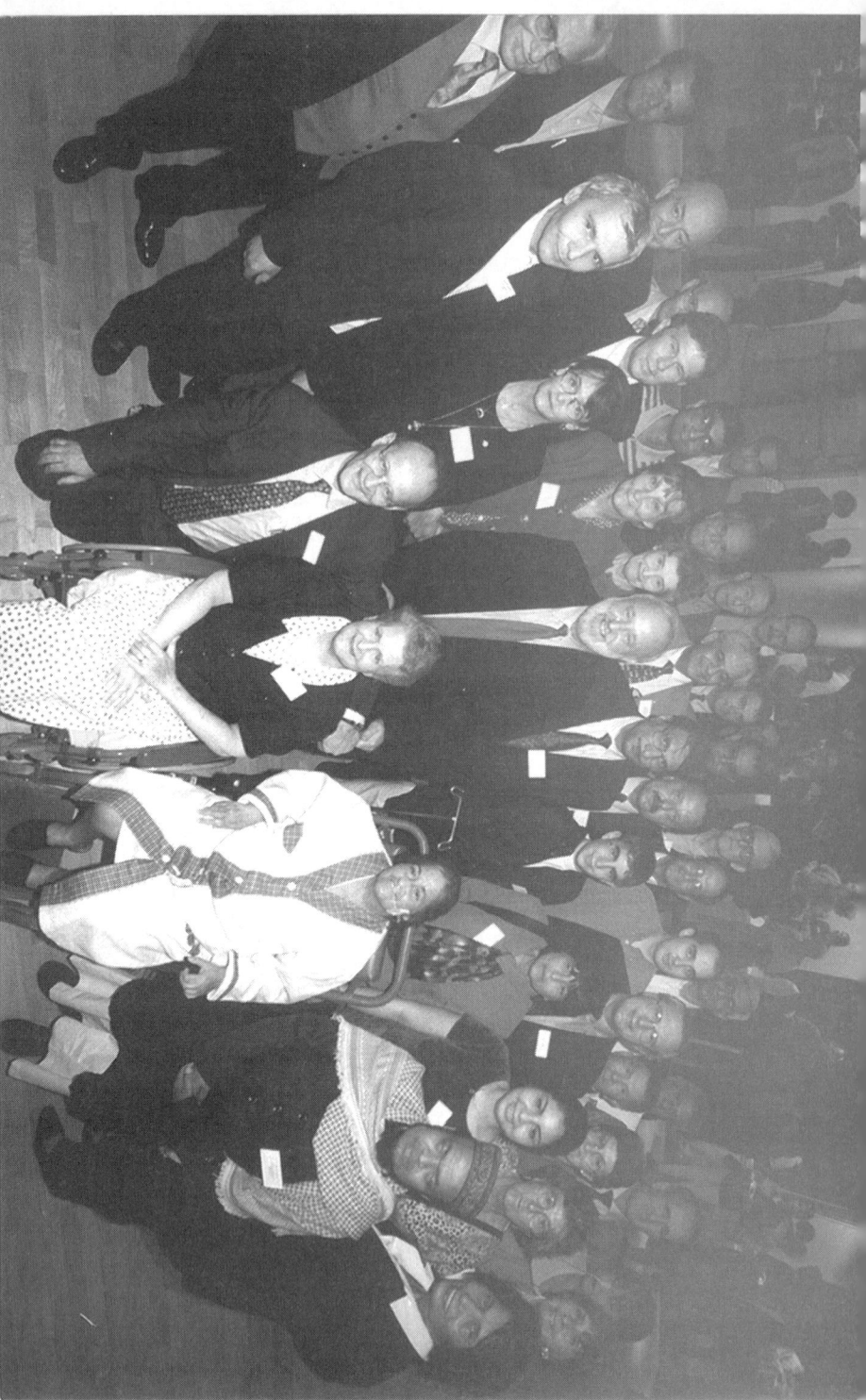

Mr. Frank Dobson, British Secretary of State for Health, Dr. A. Burroughs, Mr. K. Rolles, with liver transplant patients at celebration of 500 liver transplants, on 5th June 1998, held at the Royal Free Hospital

BOOK TWO

CARING FOR YOUR LIVER

1

Facts and Figures

Did You know that, according to the World Health Organisation (WHO) Report, published in October 1996:

*** "Hepatitis B has infected 2,000 million people around the world and;

*** There are 350 million of them are chronically infected and therefore at risk of death from liver disease, and;

*** About 100 million of them are chronically and incurably infected with Hepatitis C, and are similarly at risk",

And did you know;

*** In a fact sheet published in June 1997, the WHO estimates that "a proportion in the order of 3% of the world population has been infected with Hepatitis C Virus, and;

*** There are more than 170 million chronic carriers who are at risk of developing liver cirrhosis and/or liver cancer", and;

*** The 170 million figure is probably an underestimated figure, for several reasons, one of them is: patients do not go to see a doctor (mostly in under-developed countries) and therefore they do not know that they are ill,

And did you know;

*** To have 170 million people infected with Hepatitis C, (around 3% of the world population) mean that health authorities and politicians are facing a very serious problem.

And did you know;

*** The numbers of people who are infected with Hepatitis B and C are (almost 2.2 billion) nearly half the world population. This astronomical figure of almost 2.2 billion people are in fact infected with a serious infectious diseases, of whom 450 million developed chronic hepatitis.

And did you know;

*** The World Health Report 1996 says that: **"Hepatitis is emerging as a global health issue"**.

And did you know;

*** The number of Americans who are infected with hepatitis A, B, C is estimated by at least 300,000 each year.

*** In Britain where there is no reliable information, the number of people who are infected with hepatitis C only, is estimated by at least 250,000.

Unfortunately, according to the World Health Organisation Report: *"Despite the emergence of some 29 new diseases in the last 20 years, there is still a lack of national and international political will and resources to develop and support the systems necessary to detect them and drop their spread."*

2

Liver and its structure

The liver is known as an uncomplaining organ. It is the largest internal organ of the body. It measures approximately 30 cm (12 inches) across, and 15 cm (6 inches) in depth. It weighs about, 1.5 kg (3-4 lb.), and is located on the upper right side of the abdominal cavity, directly beneath the right lung, protected by the lower half of the rib cage.

The liver plays a vital role in regulating life processes, and it has the capacity to carry out its main functions with only a small portion in working order.

The liver has the ability to grow new liver cells if it is damaged. It has also the ability to grow to its normal size and shape if part of it is removed.

The human body depends entirely on the liver, and its functions affect our health.

The liver has a very good blood supply. It has two sources of blood supply; the hepatic artery carrying oxygenated blood from the heart, and the hepatic portal vein carrying food substances absorbed from the gut into the blood. More than a litre of blood passes through the liver every minute.

Blood leaving the liver is transported through the hepatic vein. The blood is then emptied into the inferior vena cava, and from here it is passed back to the right side of the heart, to be pumped to the lungs.

The liver is made up of two separate lobes containing sub units, made up of billions of cells arranged in vertical blocks called hepatocytes.

Also present in the blocks of cells are intricate network of tiny tubes called bile canaliculi. The canaliculi merge to form bile ducts which carry bile from the liver to the intestines.

Bile is the yellow–green liquid secreted by the liver to help the body to absorb fat, and fat soluble vitamins from the diet. If the flow of bile is reduced, or blocked as a result of a disease, the absorption of fat and vitamins A, D, E and K is impaired. Lack of vitamin D may result in brittle bones. Vitamin K is essential for blood clotting, and its deficiency causes people to bleed and bruise easily.

Functions of the liver

This complex and vital organ, is the body's chemical factory. It performs many important and complicated functions, which are vital and essential for life and maintaining good health. Some of the main functions are as follow:

1- The liver plays a key role in breaking down and converting food into useful substances for life and rapid growth of the body.

Blood that leaves the intestines must pass through the liver first. The liver is well placed to process nutrients and drugs absorbed from the digestive system, and change them into forms that are easier for the rest of the body to use. The liver can be thought of as the body's refinery.

2- The liver plays a principal role in removing any toxins and foreign substances from the blood that otherwise would be poisonous. It converts them to substances that can easily be eliminated from the body. This process is called detoxification.

3- The liver helps the body to resist and fight infections by producing immune factors. It also helps in cleaning the blood by removing bacteria from it, and discharging it as waste products into the bile. If the liver is damaged, the body's ability to fight infections is impaired.

4- The liver produces quick energy when it is needed by releasing the stored glycogen. It also manufactures new body proteins.

5- The liver helps to regulate the amount of sugar in the blood, and prevents shortages in body fuel by storing sugar, vitamins, and minerals.

6- The liver maintains hormone balance and controls the production of cholesterol.

7- The liver aids the digestive process by producing bile to digest fat in the intestine.

8- The liver destroys old red blood cells that wear out and stop working properly, (blood cells normally wear out and stop working after nearly four months of its formation). The liver then breaks them up and the unwanted haemoglobin is converted into coloured substances which pass out with the bile.

9- The liver produces heats, from the many chemical reactions that take place in the liver. As blood flows through the liver, it is warmed up and this helps to keep the body warm.

10- The liver maintain normal functions such as regulating blood clotting, fighting infection, transporting substances in the bloodstream, and hormonal balances.

3

Caring For Your Liver

Your liver is a noble and patient organ, but if it started to complain, your body will be complaining too, and your health will be seriously at risk.

Before you were born, your liver served as the main organ of blood formation. It helps your immune system to resist infections and removes bacteria from the blood stream. It keeps you, healthy all your life.

The liver, is the master organ for creating optimal nutrition for all the cells in the human body. It is probably the only organ that is most assaulted by the toxins of our modern lifestyles, that are full of pollution, stress, junk food, drugs and other dangerous chemicals.

These environmental issues together with the other social problems of our contemporary world have exposed all of us to serious health problems.

Enjoying a healthy life, depend a great deal on a healthy liver that is functioning properly.

If your liver does not perform well, its many jobs

will be affected. Whatever you eat or drink, your cells can still be grossly malnourished, if your liver does not function well.

It is your liver that transforms digested food nutrients into forms that the bloodstream can distribute to your body's cells.

A healthy liver is a matter of lifestyle, therefore if you take care of what you do and what you eat or drink, you may protect your liver for your whole life.

It is always said that "Prevention is better than cure", that is why it is important to look after your physique in order to stay healthy,

It is also essential to think of your liver as a fine, delicate organ, which can be greatly affected by your daily diet and behaviour.

Unbalanced diet and abuse of alcohol and drugs can damage your liver. Once your liver is damaged your general health will damaged too.

It is useful to remember, that: **YOUR LIVER IS A VITAL ORGAN, AND YOUR LIFE DEPENDS ON IT.**

If your liver fails to function properly, all the toxic material will find its way quite easily to the rest of your body, exposing you to danger and even to sudden death.

Your liver works twenty-four hours a day to make sure that the body's cells receives the nutrients that they need to function properly. It is not only important but it is essential, to care for your liver in order to keep yourself healthy all your life.

Caring for the liver, is a matter of common sense, and standard hygiene practice. It is very important to know more about the nutrients and materials that may cause damage to your liver, and try to avoid it.

As a guide line, the following nutrients and materials must be avoided at all times;

1- **Alcohol**, too much alcohol is largely responsible for the damage of liver, brain, heart, kidney, skin and blood vessels lining.

2- **Smoking**, while many people are aware of the negative effects of smoking on the heart and the lungs, less consideration is given to its effects on the liver. Tobacco smoke, gets into the bloodstream through the lungs, and the liver must detoxify them. All the components of smoke may cause damage to your liver.

3- **Drugs and long term drug therapy**, also over the counter medicine without consulting doctors may cause serious damages to the liver.

4- **Overheated** 'junk food,' such as french fries, fried chicken, chips, etc. These heated junk foods are a major source of toxic acids. Also some chemicals and fatty acids are causing damage to the liver cells. Some chemicals are considered to be powerfully immune suppressive, that damage liver cells.

5- **Driving** on crowded, exhaust-filled roads and highways, where the air is polluted by diesel fuels, motor oil, and gasoline, etc., are causes of liver disease. These materials are liver-toxic and may be absorbed through the skin or by inhaling them.

6- **High levels of pesticides** that are used in agriculture cause chronic liver damage.

7- **Heavy metals** such as lead, and chemicals such as solvents, sulphuric acid, paint sprays, and some cosmetic chemicals, can seriously cause damage to the liver.

These are just few examples of a long list of substances that should be avoided at all times. It offers clues as to food, drinks and materials that cause mild or chronic liver damage.

Caring for your liver

Your liver serves as the main organ of blood formation. It helps you to resist infections, removes bacteria from the blood stream, and to stay healthy.

To care for your liver you must:

1- As a golden rule, try to maintain as normal a life as possible by eating a well-balanced diet, keeping fit, and adapting a positive attitude to life. Avoid depressing or overwhelming tasks and learn how to be at peace with yourself. Rest when you feel tired. Plan some sort of physical exercise in the morning when your energy level is at its peak.

2- Never drink more than two alcoholic drinks a day.

3- Never mix medicine with alcoholic drinks.

4- Avoid taking medicine unnecessarily.

5- Make certain you have good ventilation whenever you use sprays, paints, or toxic materials. Use a mask, cover your mouth and nose, and wash off with soap and water, any chemicals that touch your skin.

6- Avoid exposure to industrial chemicals whenever possible.

7- Avoid stressful situations and learn how to relax when you are tired.

8- Maintain a healthy balanced diet and avoid processed and fatty foods.

9- Reduce the intake of refined sugars.

10- Avoid constipation by eating foods that are rich in fibres such as fresh fruit and vegetables and drink plenty of water.

11- Take regular physical exercise.

12- Learn to listen to your body, and consult your doctor if you notice any signs or symptoms of liver disease.

13- Reduce the risk of infections, by eating fresh, and clean food, and never re-heat cooked food many time.

14- Discuss being vaccinated for hepatitis A, and hepatitis B, with your doctor.

4

Eating for Healthy Liver

Everything you eat or drink, breathe and absorb through your skin must be refined by your liver. That is why considerable attention must be given to your nutrition and diet in order to keep your liver healthy.

The food you eat is broken down in your stomach and intestine, then the nutrients from the food pass through your intestine where they are absorbed into the bloodstream and transported to your liver. These elements are converted in the liver into substances the body can use.

The relation between nutrition and liver diseases is under investigation. However, good nutrition and balanced diet helps in keeping your liver healthy, and in regenerating new liver cells.

This good nutrition and balanced diet must consist of adequate amounts of carbohydrates, fats, and proteins as well as vitamins and minerals.

Healthy eating also plays an important role and sometimes is considered to be an essential part of treatment for some liver diseases.

The liver performs many unique and important metabolic tasks. It processes carbohydrates, proteins, fats and minerals to be used in maintaining normal body functions.

Carbohydrates, or glucose in our diet comes from starch and sugar. It is found in food such as bread, potatoes, fruit and sweets.

Carbohydrates are broken down in the digestive system to glucose. Any glucose not used immediately for energy is stored as glycogen in the liver and some in the muscles. The liver quickly converts glycogen back into glucose to be used when the body needs extra energy.

In this way, the liver helps to regulate the blood sugar level. It also prevents sugar from rising or falling too far. This enable us to keep an even level of energy throughout the day.

Fat, is a very important element in our daily diet. It comes from butter, cheese, cooking oil, animal fat and from many 'invisible' sources, such as biscuits, pastries, and cakes.

Fat cannot be digested without bile, which is made in the liver and stored in the gallbladder. Bile is released when needed into the small intestine and acts as a detergent, breaking fat into tiny droplets so that it can be absorbed by the body. Bile is also essential for the absorption of vitamins A, D, E, and K.

Fats are a useful source of calories and provides fat soluble vitamins A, D, E, and K and essential fatty acids. So a person who restricts fat in their diet should try to eat extra carbohydrate, such as starch and sugar (for example bread and honey).

Protein, comes in our diet from food such as

meat, fish, eggs, cheese and nuts. Protein is made up of units called amino acids. When these acids reach the liver they are either released to the muscles as energy, stored for later use, or converted to urea for excretion in the urine. The liver has a unique ability to convert some amino acids into sugar for quick energy.

In the past, liver treatment has included a low protein diet. Now it is realised that restricting protein is unnecessary and harmful. This is because it contributes to malnutrition and weakness. Low protein diets are not recommended except in some rare situations in severely ill people in hospital.

Balanced and Healthy Diet:

Good nutrition, and balanced diet can help the damaged liver to regenerate new liver cells.

Poor nutrition, can affect the liver and may take the blame for some liver diseases. It is thought that many chronic liver diseases are associated in one way or another with malnutrition.

Eating for healthy liver, good nutrition and diet should contain sufficient protein, low in fat, sugar, and salt. It should also contain high fibre and wide range of vitamins and minerals.

Healthy eating means getting the right balance between different foods. A diet that includes lots of vegetables, fruit, beans, and wholemeal cereals (including bread) and is low in fat, is considered to be a good diet for many people who suffer from liver disease.

Vitamins and Minerals:

Our bodies need a variety of vitamins and minerals. They are essential for the chemical reactions which occur in our bodies every day. They enable our bodies to carry out all the processes necessary for life.

Most people get all the vitamins and minerals their bodies need by choosing a variety of foods from the following food groups:
  A- bread, cereal, potatoes, rice, pasta
  B- fruit and vegetables
  C- milk, yoghurt, eggs, and cheese
  D- meat, fish, nuts, and beans

It is important to choose every day a variety of food from these groups in order to get a balanced diet. However, you must remember:
  1- To eat plenty of raw fruits and vegetables, they are high in the fibre that you need and also prevent constipation.
  2- To chew food thoroughly.
  3- To eat fresh food and to avoid eating junk food or re-heated food for more than twice.
  4- To avoid excessively saturated or damaged fats.
  5- To have breakfast with cereal served with milk.
  6- To avoid eating large amounts of sugar, and you must remember that the liver converts sugar into fat.
  7- To drink at least ten to twelve glasses of water a day. This helps to clean your liver and kidneys.
  8- To make your meal time pleasurable, and try not to eat if you are upset or depressed.

Some Eating Problems:
Some people, especially those who suffer from liver diseases, find eating a well balanced diet is difficult.

This can happen sometimes because many liver patients experience either loss of appetite or nausea, or both. For instance people with cirrhosis require a balanced diet, rich in protein, but because of their illness they do not feel like eating at all. However, it is important for them to eat as well as possible. British

Liver Trust published a booklet, 'Diet and liver disease,' giving advice on how to tackle these problems.

The following are some tips that may help you:

Loss of appetite:
* Eat small but frequent meals, little and often.
* nutritious snacks may be better than a big meal.
* Try to eat something every two hours, however small.
* Tempt yourself with foods that you like.
* Do not force yourself to eat foods you do not like.
* Try to relax before and after you eat.
* Take your time over eating, chew well and breathe steadily.
* If you do not feel like eating solid food, try to have a nourishing drink instead.

Nausea:
* Some smells make you feel sick, in that case, try a breath of fresh air before you eat.
* Keep your mouth fresh by brushing your teeth, using a mouthwash or sucking mints.
* Do not let yourself to go hungry for too long.
* Try to eat five or more small meals instead of two or three big meals.
* Cold snacks may be better tolerated than a hot main meals.
* Avoid eating when you are tired, relax first.

No salt diet:
* Avoid all salt added at the table.
* Avoid stock cubes, and gravy granules.
* Avoid packet and tinned soups, tinned vegetables including baked beans.
* Avoid smoked and tinned fish, including salmon, tuna and pilchards.

* Avoid cured fish and meats, including ham, bacon, sausages.

* Avoid cheese, except cottage cheese and cream cheese.

* Avoid all bottled sauces and ketchup.

5

Liver Diseases

Liver diseases appear to be on the increase. Part of this increase may be due to our frequent contact with chemicals and environmental pollutants.

The amount of medicines and other drugs consumed by people has increased greatly in the last fifty years. As a result the liver has been exposed to many poisonous materials, and that lead in turn to liver diseases.

However, there are many types and kinds of liver diseases and liver damage but the most common diseases are: hepatitis, alcohol related disorder, cirrhosis, liver disorder in children and cancer of the liver. These are most serious liver diseases.

Statistics show that hepatitis, which is caused by several viruses that attack and infect the liver is the most common of liver diseases.

Nevertheless, the symptoms of most liver diseases, as well as hepatitis, are similar but differ slightly. This is due to the causes of the original disease.

It all begins with a vague feeling of ill health, and the liver often becomes tender and enlarged. However patients usually exhibit one or two of the following symptoms in the early stage of the disease.

Signs and Symptoms of Liver Disease

The main symptoms of liver diseases vary slightly, however people who observe any of the following symptoms or signs should consult their doctors immediately.

1- Jaundice (Yellow colour of the eyes and skin), in many cases is the first, and is sometimes the only sign of liver disease.

2- An increasing feeling of fatigue, apathy and loss of stamina.

3- Tendency to bleed or bruise easily.

4- Prolonged itching.

5- Dark coloured urine and pale, yellow, or light-coloured stools.

6- Bleeding, nausea or Vomiting of blood, or passing of bloody or dark stools.

7- Abdominal swelling, and abdominal pain. Liver disease may cause ascites, which is an accumulation of fluid in the abdominal cavity.

8- Loss of appetite, and unusual change in weight, (increase or decrease in weight)

9- Loss of sexual drive or performance.

10- Sleep disturbances, mental confusion and coma, are present in severe liver disease. These symptoms are the result of an accumulation of toxic substances in the body that impair the brain function.

11- Failure to grow normally in young children.

What Is Hepatitis?

Hepatitis is the most common and serious liver disease. The word, hepatitis, means literary any inflammation of the liver. It is derived from the Greek word for liver, hepar. It is commonly described as either acute or chronic liver disease.

The most common cause of hepatitis is viral

infection of the liver, caused by several different viruses. However, there are other causes of hepatitis that are non viral, such as alcohol, chemical agents or poisons; drugs; bacteria or bacterial toxins; amoebic disease; and certain parasitic infestations.

Hepatitis can progress to a chronic state that may in turn lead to cirrhosis. This is another serious liver disease and when it becomes severe, it destroys the liver cells.

There are different types of hepatitis viruses such as, hepatitis A, B, C, D, E. and G. The main different between all of them is in the way that they are spread and the effects that they have on the patient's health. The three most common viruses are, hepatitis A, hepatitis B and hepatitis C.

HEPATITIS A (HAV)

Hepatitis A virus, is also called infectious or epidemic hepatitis. It is a relatively mild infection, though it can lead to coma and death especially among older people.

It affects people of all ages, but it is most common among children especially in developing countries. It is also common between adults in the developed countries.

Hepatitis A, is very common in many countries in southern and eastern Europe, Africa and the Middle and Far East. The number of people who are infected in the UK is relatively low, but this is likely to be under estimated since there are many people with mild symptoms of hepatitis A, who never consult their doctor.

Hepatitis A virus, spreads through contaminated water and food, and is excreted in the stool. It is also spreading because of poor personal hygiene in areas of poor sanitation and contaminated drinking water supplies with sewage disposal. Infection can be easily spread by direct contact with an infected person.

It is also more common between homosexual communities, and injection drug users. There is also a rare risk of transmission via blood transfusions or other blood products.

The severity of the disease increases with age and there is a small risk of death, particularly in people over the age of sixty years old. In infants and young children the infection can be mild or even unnoticed.

Symptoms of Hepatitis A

Some people may have no symptoms at all, but they can still be infected and unknowingly pass on the virus. Others may develop a serious illness.

There is an incubation period of between two to six weeks before symptoms develop. The most common symptoms can include, headache, fever, nausea and vomiting, abdominal pain and diarrhoea.

These symptoms may last for a week or more before jaundice develops. Jaundice is easily noticeable as the skin and whites of the eyes turn yellow, the urine turns dark and stools become pale.

Prevention

Hepatitis A infection is largely preventable by good hygiene. It can also be prevented by vaccination which provides protection for up to ten years. Short term protection can be provided by a single injection of immunoglobulin which lasts for about three to six months. Protection is recommended for people who have been in close contact with hepatitis A patients, or for travellers to areas where the infection is more widespread.

HEPATITIS B (HBV)

Hepatitis B, is also known as hep. B, or serum hepatitis. It is caused by hepatitis B virus. It is generally more serious than hepatitis A. It is the most common form of hepatitis, with around 350 million infected patients around the world. It often becomes chronic and may lead to cirrhosis, even to liver cancer, and eventually liver failure occurs.

Some people may be ill for a few weeks and then recover completely. Others because the initial symptoms of hepatitis B may not be severe, may never realise that they have been infected, until the liver has already been damaged.

A few people carry the virus all their lives, and some of them may develop symptoms of liver disease, whilst others have no symptoms and may be unaware that they are infected.

Hepatitis B, virus is spread by contact with infected blood, saliva, semen, and other body fluids, as well as through blood transfusion.

The virus is mainly transmitted through blood to blood contact. This means that a small amount of blood from one person who carries the virus can spread the infection if it gets into someone else's bloodstream.

Infection can result, for example, from unprotected sex with an infected person or accidental injury with a contaminated needle. Injection drug users who share needles and other injecting equipment have a high risk of infection.

It can be transmitted through cuts or by simple acts such as kissing, ear piercing, tattooing or even dental work carried out with equipment that has not been sterilised properly. It can also be transmitted from a pregnant woman to her child.

Hepatitis B is very common in some parts of the world such as South east Asia, the Middle and Far East, Southern Europe and Africa.

The World Health Organisation (WHO), estimates that one third of the world's population has been infected with hepatitis B, and that there are around 350 million chronically infected people world-wide.

In Europe there are estimated to be one million people infected every year. In the UK approximately one in 1,000 people carry the virus.

The majority of adults who are infected with hepatitis B, recover fully. Less than ten per cent became chronically infected. The continuing liver inflammation and damage caused by long term infection may lead to cirrhosis and liver cancer. People who develop cirrhosis need careful monitoring by a specialist in liver diseases.

Symptoms of Hepatitis B

There is an incubation period of between six weeks to six months before any symptoms may appear. However, many people never have any symptoms, and do not feel ill although they are still infected.

Whenever there are symptoms, some people notice a mild, 'flu like illness' that may include a cough, sore throat, tiredness, joint pains and loss of appetite. Some other people may have nausea and vomiting. Occasionally an acute infection can be severe, with abdominal pain and jaundice.

People most at risk of infection are, injection drug users, babies born to infected mothers, close family members and partners of an infected person, health-care workers who have direct contact with blood - doctors, dentists, nurses and midwives, prisoners, people travelling and working in countries where the virus is endemic.

Protection

Because of the danger from hepatitis B, a vaccine against it is recommended. Three injections of the vaccine are needed for full protection. The first injection is followed by the second one a month later and another at six months.

Babies can be protected by vaccination at birth if it is known that the mother is a carrier.

In the USA vaccination against hepatitis B is strongly recommended for those who are exposed to body fluids as well as for young children. Unfortunately, vaccination for hepatitis B has not been strongly recommended in the UK.

Prof. A. J. Zuckerman, the Principal and Dean of the school of Medicine at the Royal Free Hospital, wrote in a 'Letter to the Editor,' The Times Newspaper, saying that: *"In 1992 the World Health Organisation recommended the introduction of universal immunisation of infants and/or adolescents by 1997, and some 95 countries, including most European countries, have now implemented its recommendation. It would surly be appropriate for the UK to protect the nation against this infection on the 50th anniversary of the NHS".*

HEPATITIS C (HCV)

Hepatitis C, formerly called non-A, non B hepatitis. The virus is mainly transmitted through blood to blood contact, and it causes inflammation of the liver.

Hepatitis C virus, is one of the more recently discovered of hepatitis viruses. It was discovered in 1988, and doctors are learning more about the virus all the time.

Injection drug users and people who have had blood transfusions in the UK prior to September 1991 are most at risk. The screening of donated blood for all viruses including hepatitis, started in the UK in September 1991.

The prevalence of hepatitis C, world-wide is largely unknown because most people have no symptoms. The

Call for protection from hepatitis B

From Professor A. J. Zuckerman

Sir, The recent outbreak of hepatitis B in Devon (reports, July 21 and 22) serves to remind us that more than a third of the world population has been infected with this virus. There are thought to be 350 million chronic carriers (not all of them infectious) and the virus is estimated to result in between one and two million deaths annually worldwide; each year one million people are infected in the European region alone.

Nearly half of all cases contract the infection by the sexual route, rather than by blood-to-blood contact, and all sexually active individuals (heterosexual and homosexual) are at an increased risk. Intravenous drug abuse with unsterile equipment is also a major risk, accounting for up to 35 per cent of acute hepatitis B in the US, Denmark, Sweden and Switzerland.

It is unlikely that the UK differs statistically from the rest of Europe. Figures from unselective screening of pregnant women in the West Midlands, for example, revealed that while carriers were uncommon among Caucasian women, prevalence among women attending antenatal clinics from the Indian sub-continent was one in 100, one in 140 among Afro-Caribbeans and one in 14 among Chinese women (South East Asia and the Far East).

In 1992 the World Health Organisation recommended the introduction of universal immunisation of infants and/or adolescents by 1997, and some 95 countries, including most European countries, have now implemented its recommendation. It would surely be appropriate for the UK to protect the nation against this infection on the 50th anniversary of the NHS.

Yours etc,
A. J. ZUCKERMAN
(Principal and Dean),
Royal Free Hospital

World Health Organisation (WHO), estimates that 3% of the world's population has HCV and that 200 million people world-wide are chronically infected.

Hepatitis C, affects approximately 170,000 American each year. Large number of these people may develop chronic liver disease and cirrhosis.

A high percentage of people with chronic hepatitis C, do not know how they caught it. The exact sources of infection are still unclear. However, infection is not thought to be picked up through normal social contact, and also it is still unknown whether hepatitis C can be transmitted sexually.

It is estimated that, currently around 80 per cent of patients who have contracted hepatitis C virus, have failed to clear the virus and may go on to develop chronic hepatitis and that can lead to cirrhosis of the liver or even cancer.

Chronic hepatitis C

Chronic hepatitis C, refers to infections that do not clear up within six months after the initial infection. The liver remains inflamed and gradually destroys the normal cells, causing damage to the liver cells itself.

The disease may gradually progress over a period of ten to forty years. A liver biopsy can identify the type and degree of the damage and can determine the severity of the disease. It is believed that more than 20 per cent of the patients with chronic hepatitis C will develop cirrhosis.

Symptoms of hepatitis C

Hepatitis C virus can effect people in many different ways. The majority of people who are already infected with hepatitis C, do not have serious symptoms, or have no symptoms at all. Many of them are often unaware they have been infected.

Others may develop symptoms such as, extreme tiredness and often feel unwell. Symptoms of hepatitis C, may be vague, however, it may include: Mild to severe fatigue, anxiety weight loss, joint pains, pain in the area of the liver, concentration problems, nausea, loss of appetite fever, headaches, and abdominal pain, and sometimes diarrhoea.

Vaccines are available to prevent infection from hepatitis A, and B viruses, but unfortunately it is not from hepatitis C, up till now.

HEPATITIS D (HDV)

Formerly called delta virus or hepatitis D. People who are infected with hepatitis B, also have hepatitis D virus. Being infected with both viruses is known as co-infection and usually results in more severe liver disease. It is transmitted in blood in the same way as in hepatitis B. It is most common among injection drug users.

HEPATITIS E (HEV)

Formerly called epidemic non-A, non-B hepatitis. It is spread in the same way as in hepatitis A virus. Both viruses are excreted or shed in faeces. It is transmitted by direct contact with an infected person's faeces, or indirect faecal contamination of food, and water supply.

CIRRHOSIS

Cirrhosis of the liver is a degenerative disease where liver cells are damaged and replaced by scar formation. As scar tissue progressively accumulates, blood flow through the liver is diminished, causing even more liver cells to die, and the patient may die of liver failure.

Cirrhosis is a serious liver disease, that resulted

from a long term of continuous liver damage. It is associated in most cases with drinking too much alcohol, combined with a poor diet. However, this is not always the case.

In general, cirrhosis can be associated with anything that results in severe liver injury, such as long term infection with hepatitis. It is reported that over half of the deaths from cirrhosis are caused by excessive consumption of alcohol, hepatitis and infections.

Some chemicals, many poisons, too much iron or copper, severe reaction to drugs, and obstruction of the bile duct can also cause cirrhosis. If cirrhosis is advanced, people may develop many complications such as ascites, bleeding and some other complications caused by the waste products that are normally broken down by the liver, which in turn enter the blood circulation and affect the brain.

Ascites is a large build up of fluid in the abdomen, and bleeding is caused by the increase of blood pressure in the veins.

At this point, treatment is mostly supportive and may include a strict diet, diuretics, vitamins, and abstinence from alcohol.

However, there has been much progress in managing the major complications of cirrhosis such as fluid retention in the abdomen, bleeding, and changes in mental function.

Each year over 25,000 Americans die from cirrhosis, the seventh leading cause of death in the United States of America.

CANCER OF LIVER

The most common forms of cancer of the liver begin in other parts of the body and spread to the liver. However, there are some other forms of cancer that originate in the liver which are associated with viral hepatitis and certain parasites, drug, and environmental toxin. Chronic carriers of the hepatitis B or C viruses are at risk of developing liver cancer.

Very little is known about cancer that originates in the liver except that it is associated with viral hepatitis, certain parasites, and environmental toxins. Each year, 1,000 Americans die of primary liver cancer.

ALCOHOL-RELATED LIVER DISEASES

Almost everyone who drinks excessive amounts of alcohol will get some liver disorder related to alcohol such as fatty liver, alcoholic hepatitis, and alcoholic cirrhosis.

Fatty liver, is the most common alcohol-related liver disorder. It causes enlargement of the liver and right upper abdominal discomfort. The swollen liver is often tender or painful. Severe fatty liver may cause temporary jaundice and abnormalities of liver function. An abstinence from alcohol may cure without leaving residual cirrhosis.

Alcoholic hepatitis is an acute illness often characterised by nausea, vomiting, right upper and middle abdominal pain, fever, jaundice, enlarged and tender liver, and an elevation of the white blood cell count. Sometimes alcoholic hepatitis may be present without symptoms. As with fatty liver, treatment is primarily supportive and preventive.

Once alcoholic hepatitis develops, progression to cirrhosis will occur if alcohol consumption continues.

Alcoholic cirrhosis occurs in ten to fifteen per cent of people who consume large amounts of alcohol over a prolonged period of time. However, there is considerable variation in the degree of susceptibility of people to given amounts of alcohol, and further research is needed to determine why some individuals are more vulnerable to alcohol than others.

However, any disease which is brought on by alcohol abuse cannot be reversed until alcohol intake is stopped.

LIVER DISORDERS IN CHILDREN

Tens of thousands of American children, from new born infants to adolescents, get liver diseases, and hundreds of these children die every year from them.

There are more than 100 different types of liver diseases that have been identified in infants and children.

COMMON LIVER DISORDERS IN CHILDREN

Biliary Atresia

Is caused by the absence or an inadequate size of bile ducts from the liver to the intestine that is unable to excrete bile. The infant usually dies from cirrhosis and bleeding by the age of two years. A surgical operation may relieve obstruction in a small percentage of cases.

Chronic Active Hepatitis

Gradually destroys and replaces the normal liver cells with scar tissue through an unknown process that resembles an allergy to the child's own liver tissue.

6

Liver Transplantation

The first liver transplant operation in the world, was performed in the USA, in 1963 by professor Thomas Starzl in Denver.

The first liver transplant in the UK was performed in 1968 by Professor Sir Roy Calne at Addenbrookes Hospital, Cambridge.

However, the procedure of liver transplantation did not gain widespread acceptance in medical practice until the 1980's.

At the Royal Free Hospital, a liver transplant programme started in 1988, and is now firmly established as one of the leading liver transplant centres in the world.

Liver transplantation has become the only treatment for most patients with chronic liver diseases and acute liver failure that were one day threatening their lives.

Nevertheless, because cancers of the liver begin somewhere else in the body, and spread to the liver, transplantation cannot be considered as an form of treatment for many cases of liver cancers. However, some medical bodies believe that transplantation at an early stage of liver cancer, may result in long-term survival for some patients.

In adults, liver transplantation is considered to be the best, or perhaps the only form of treatment for liver cirrhosis, death of liver cells. In children, a biliary atresia, a failure of the bile ducts to develop normally to drain bile from the liver, are the diseases that are most often treated by liver transplantation.

However, some patients who develop cirrhosis of the liver due to excessive use of alcohol do not need liver transplantation. Abstinence from alcohol and treatment of complications may allow them to live for prolonged periods without a liver transplantation.

Before doctors can decide whether liver transplantation is the best form of treatment, it is necessary to have a pre-transplant assessment. This assessment consists of a series of medical tests designed to study the extent of the disease in the liver and to give a thorough picture of the overall health condition of the patient. They are also designed to help doctors and the rest of the transplant team to do everything possible to assure a successful transplant.

Once a patient has completed all the necessary tests and investigations and the doctors are satisfied with the result, the patient will be registered with the United Kingdom Transplant Services (UKTS) in Bristol. Name and details are added to the waiting list and the transplant assistants will give the patient a bleeper to facilitate the contact with the patient.

In any case it is important that liver transplant patients and their families must understand the risks that are involved with proceeding to the liver transplantation.

Nevertheless, improvements in surgical

techniques and immunosuppressive therapy have led to steady increase in the survival of liver transplant patients.

The average waiting time for liver transplantation is between six to eight weeks, although it may vary depending on blood group and weight. There is no numerical order of priority on the waiting list, each person is assessed individually and the most suitable patient will have the priority.

In liver transplantation, the patient has been given a new liver from another person. The body recognises that this new organ is a 'foreign' body, and try to reject and attack it.

Immunosuppressive therapy can help to suppress the immune system and to stop attacking the newly transplanted liver and protect it from being rejected. That is why it is very important that liver transplant patients must take the anti-rejection drugs regularly and exactly as doctors recommend.

The overall chances of surviving a liver transplant are on the increase, and now the survival rate is very high indeed. That was due to the new invention of the immunosuppressive therapy (anti-rejection drugs).

When the first liver transplantation was performed, Prednisolone, was used to block some of the cells that trigger a rejection response. This is a steroid drug that is used immediately after the transplantation. It has many serious undesirable side effects.

However, since the discovery of Cyclosporine in the eighties, liver transplantation is considered today to be a successful treatment. Cyclosporine is one of these drugs that has been used by liver transplant patients for over ten years now. It helps to prevent the body from rejecting the transplanted liver. It was the most important ingredient for the success of liver transplantation. The dosage of cyclosporin is adjusted according to the patient's weight, liver and kidney functions. It is also adjusted according to the level of cyclosporin in the blood.

However, because of its side effects, leading drug companies never stop searching for a better immunosuppressive therapy, even though real breakthroughs are rare in this field.

The discovery of Tacrolimus (Prograf capsules) or FK 506 was considered to be a real breakthrough for liver transplant patients. It works in the same way as Cyclosporin, but it is thought to have less side effects and it may suit liver transplant patients better.

Mycophenolate mofetil (CellCept) is another new anti-rejection medication. It was discovered in the mid nineties and it was initially used to be given to kidney transplant patients. However, liver specialist tried it with liver transplant patients and found it useful particularly with patients who are suffering from kidney trouble.

The amalgamation of skills and medical hi-technology have provided physicians and surgeons with the right ingredients of successful transplant operations. However, with transplantation there are risks common to all forms of major surgery, as well as technical difficulties in removing the diseased liver and implanting the donor's liver.

One of the major risks for the patients is not having any liver function for a brief period. Immediately after surgery, bleeding, poor function of the new liver, and infections are major risks.

Before going to the operating theatre patients will receive some pre-medication that make them feel sleepy and relaxed.

During the transplantation, frequent tests are done to monitor the liver functions and detect any evidence of rejection.

After the transplant operation, the patient will be

taken directly to the Intensive Care Unit (ICU), where they will be looked after by doctors and nurses who are specifically trained and experienced in this speciality. The transplant team will also be involved in the care that the patient receives in the Intensive Care Unit.

In the Intensive Care Unite, the patients will be very sleepy and nurses will be monitoring their hearts, blood pressure, breathing etc., all the time to make sure that the patients are comfortable.

Initially in the intensive care unit, the body functions including the liver of any transplant patient are carefully monitored. Once the patient is transferred to the ward, the frequency of blood testing is decreased. Food is allowed and physiotherapy is used to regain patient's muscle strength. The drug or drugs that are recommended to prevent rejection are initially given through the vein, and later by mouth.

Rejection is a normal reaction of the body to the new liver. It does not mean that the transplant is failing.

In liver transplantation, rejection is less of a problem than with heart, lung, or kidney transplants. It is recorded that few liver transplant patients have very severe rejection.

Episodes of rejection are treated with larger doses of steroids that are given through an intravenous drip, once a day, for three days. Other medications may be required.

The chances of surviving a liver transplantation have improved dramatically in recent years. Today, liver transplantation has been accepted, as the most effective means of rapidly reviving the liver functions in patients with acute liver failure.

Most patients return to a full and active life and only need to take few anti-rejection medication every day to remain healthy. In general a complete recovery depends on how ill the individual patient was prior to surgery.

However, the lack of donors is the major problem that is facing liver transplantation. Research is going on at present to use primates as an alternative to human organs.

QUESTIONS
AND
ANSWERS

1

On Hepatitis

What is hepatitis?
Hepatitis is an inflammation of the liver. There are two kinds of hepatitis, viral hepatitis, transmitted by different types of viruses that attack the liver and cause inflammation, and non-viral hepatitis that is caused by substances such as chemicals, drugs and alcohol.

Viral hepatitis is caused by at least five types of viruses: hepatitis A, B, C, D, and E.

What are the causes of hepatitis A (HAV)?
Hepatitis A, is also called infectious hepatitis and is most common amongst children in developing countries. It is caused by eating contaminated food and drinking contaminated water.

What are the symptoms of hepatitis A?
There are many common symptoms, that include: fever, fatigue, loss of appetite, nausea, vomiting, pain

in the liver area, dark urine, light-coloured stools, diarrhoea and yellowing of the skin and eyes.

How is hepatitis A spread?

Hepatitis A virus is spread from one person to another in areas of poor sanitation. Infection is spread by: close personal contact with someone infected with hepatitis A, and food or water supplies contaminated with hepatitis A virus. It is also transmitted by faecal-oral route. Transmission can also be through blood transfusion or sharing needles with infected people using injectable drugs.

Is there any vaccination against hepatitis A virus?

Yes, there is a vaccination for hepatitis A virus and it is recommended for all children over two years of age. However, hepatitis A is largely preventable by practicing, good standard, sensible and sound hygiene.

What are the causes of hepatitis B?

Hepatitis B is generally a more serious liver disease, often becoming chronic. It is caused by the hepatitis B virus that infects the liver. It is estimated that around 50 million people world-wide are contracting hepatitis B annually.

Hepatitis B virus is spread by direct contact with infected blood, saliva, semen and other body fluids, as well as through blood transfusions, sharing an intravenous drug, or ear-piercing needle, and unprotected sexual intercourse. The virus can also be transmitted from mothers to babies at birth.

What are the symptoms of hepatitis B?

The common symptoms include: Fatigue; pain in muscles, joint, stomach, diarrhoea, vomiting, together with the rest of hepatitis A symptoms.

Hepatitis B is highly endemic in Africa, Southeast Asia, the Middle East, and the southern and western Pacific Islands.

Is there any vaccination against hepatitis B virus?

Yes, there is a vaccination against hepatitis B. It has been available since 1982 and is strongly recommended universally to everyone in all the countries of the world. However, some countries still do not strongly recommend vaccination to everyone. Some other countries, only recommended vaccination against hepatitis B for people who are in direct contact with high risk people. The number of people who have received the vaccine is estimated at only 500 million persons world-wide.

Is the hepatitis B vaccine safe?

Hepatitis B vaccines have been known to be very safe. The most common side effects from hepatitis B vaccinations are pain at the injection site and mild fever.

What are the causes of hepatitis C?

Hepatitis C virus is another virus that infects the liver. It is made up of a group of similar viruses that are structurally different from hepatitis B virus. Infection with hepatitis C usually occurs in adulthood. Statistics show that the majority of the people infected with hepatitis C virus are unable to treat it with medication. It normally develops to cirrhosis.

Hepatitis C is a very slow growing virus, and it may take 20 years or even more for the infected person to develop any symptoms of the disease. The causes of hepatitis C are still unknown, however, it is thought to be from the abuse of alcohol, drugs or both.

How is hepatitis C transmitted?

Hepatitis C virus was discovered in blood in the mid-1970s, however, it is not clear whether it can be transmitted through direct contact with infected blood, semen or saliva. Nevertheless, doctors advise people to take great care in handling anything that may have contaminated blood, and to have adequate protection before they expose themselves to any direct contact with body fluids.

What are the symptoms of hepatitis C?

Most people who are infected with hepatitis C have no symptoms at all. However, because the virus is in the blood it can damage the liver cells, and symptoms begin to appear only after the liver has been damaged.

If symptoms are presented, they may be flu-like symptoms, nausea, fatigue, loss of appetite, fever, headaches and abdominal pain.

Is there any vaccination against Hepatitis C virus?

Unfortunately there is no vaccination against hepatitis C yet.

What is hepatitis D (HDV)?

Hepatitis D is a blood borne virus and can only be caught by patients who already have hepatitis B. It spreads and is transmitted in the same way as hepatitis B.

What is hepatitis E (HEV)?

Hepatitis E is similar to hepatitis A. It spreads and is transmitted in exactly the same way as hepatitis A.

2

On Liver transplantation

Is liver transplantation a treatment of the last resort, when everything else has failed?

Yes, and no. If there is any other medical treatment that is likely to allow prolonged survival with good quality of life, transplantation would be reserved for the future.

Frequently medical treatment delays, but does not eliminate, the need for transplantation.

However, ideally the surgery is undertaken before the final stage of the disease, when the person is too ill to withstand major surgery and will not survive until a suitable donor is available.

How the decision is made to transplant?

The decision is made in consultation with all individuals involved in the patient's care, including the patient and the family. The patient and family's input are vital and they must clearly understand the risks that are involved with proceeding to transplantation.

What are the major risks that involved with

What are the major risks that involved with liver transplantation?

Before surgery, the risks are mainly the development of some acute complications of the disease that might render the patient unacceptable for the transplantation.

With transplantation there are risks common to all forms of major surgery, as well as technical difficulties in removing the diseased liver and implanting the donor's liver. One of the major risks for the patient is not having any liver function for a brief period.

Immediately after surgery, bleeding, poor function of the grafted liver, and infections are major risks. The patient is carefully monitored for several weeks for any sign of rejection or infection of the liver.

What are the overall chances of surviving a liver transplant?

This depends on many factors but, in general around 60-75% of the adult patients, and 80-90% of the children survive the transplantation and are discharged from the hospital. There is every indication that those who are well after one year remain so indefinitely.

How long does it take to recover?

This depends on how ill the individual was prior to the transplantation. Most patients should count on spending a few days in an intensive care unit and about two to four weeks in hospital.

If the transplanted liver fails to function, or is rejected, what can be done?

There are varying degrees of failure of the liver. However, even with imperfect function, the patient will remain quite well. Occasionally, when circumstances and time permit, a failing transplanted liver can be replaced by a second (or even third) transplant.

Do recipients of liver transplant have to take anti-rejection medicines for the rest of their lives?

Usually, yes. However, as the body adjusts to the transplanted liver, the amount of medicine needed to control rejection is reduced, There are patients who have been successfully taken off these drugs. Researchers are attempting to determine why this has been successful in these cases.

Routine follow-up consists of blood tests, measuring of blood pressure with annual or semi-annual check-ups at the transplant centre is very important to monitor the progress of the transplanted liver inside the body.

Recipients should avoid exposure to infections as the immune system is depressed. Illness should be reported to the doctor immediately and medicines taken only under medical supervision.

How long does it take the patient to regain his or her physical activity after the transplantation?

Most patients are able to return to a normal or near normal existence and can participate in fairly vigorous physical exercise six to twelve months after a successful liver transplant. As with other physical activities, sexual activity may be resumed.

Is it safe for women to become pregnant after transplantation?

Studies have shown that women who undergo liver transplantation can conceive and give birth normally, although they have to be monitored carefully because of a higher incidence of premature births.

What about patient's diet?
Transplant patients have a tendency to gain weight because of their retention of water. They are advised to lower their intake of salt to reduce or eliminate this water retention. Otherwise patients should maintain a balanced diet.

Glossary

Glossary

Acyclovir: A drug that is used to prevent or to treat viruses such as herpes simplex. It is used with patients whose immune systems are disturbed and when patients have lower resistance to infection due to medication or disease.

Amphotericin: An antibiotic that is used to treat infection of the mouth and gut, during the first few months of the transplanted organ.

Angiocardiogram: An X-ray examination is performed after a dye is injected directly into the a blood vessel in the groin by means of a slim sterile flexible tube. It is used to show the arteries and veins, their contours, and any narrowing or blockage that may be an important consideration during any surgery.

Antidiuretic hormone (ADH): A hormone released by pituitary gland, that increases the re-absorption of water by the kidney and preventing excessive loss of water from the body.

Ascites: An accumulation of fluid in the peritoneal cavity causes abdominal swelling. It can make the abdomen so distended that patients look as if they are pregnant. It is very uncomfortable, making breathing and eating difficult.

Azathioprine (Imuran): An anti-rejection drug used to prevent rejection of a transplanted organ.

Biliary atresia: A liver condition common in young children, result from an absence or inadequate size of bile duct in which the bile ducts do not drain. Some forms of biliary atresia can be corrected surgically, but if diagnosis has been delay the condition may lead to irreversible liver damage.

Bile Ducts: The channels that convey bile from the liver. Bile is drained from the liver cells by many small ducts that unite to form the main bile duct of the liver.

Bone scan: an x-ray to assess the condition of the bones.

CellCept (mycophenolate mofetil): A new powerful immunosuppressive drug (anti-rejection) used to prevent the body from rejecting the transplanted organ.

Cirrhosis: A condition in which the liver cells are damaged and repaced by fibres that grow in the liver.

C.T.Scan: (computerized tomography) a computerizes X-ray examination in which the x-ray source and the detector rotate around the liver to produce a good picture of the liver that shows its size and shape and major blood vessels.

Colonoscopy: A medical procedure in which a flexible fibre-optic is passed into back passage to assess the condition of the colon.

Cyclosporin (Sadimmun/Neoral): A drug that suppresses the immune system to prevent the body from rejecting the transplanted organ. There are tow forms of cyclosporin, Sandimmun and Neoral.

Didronel: A drug that is used to treat various disorders of the bone metabolism, and in combination with calcium is used to treat osteoporosis.

Electrocardiogram (ECG): A medical test recording the electrical activity of the heart to determine any abnormality especially signs of the coronary heart disease. The recording is done while a patient is walking on a treadmill or ride a stationary bicycle.

Echocardiogram: This procedure uses sound waves to assess the heart function and is done immediately prior the ECG.

Electroencephalogram (EEG): A medical test that is used for recording the electrical activity in the brain that may occur with liver disease. Tiny wires or electrodes are attached to the scalp with a special gel.

Endoscopy: A medical procedure performed under sedation, in which a flexible fibre-optic tube is passed through the mouth into the oesophagus and stomach to check for enlarged veins (varices) which are often the result of prolonged liver disease.

Endoscopic Retrograde Cholaniopancreatgraphy (ERCP): Medical procedure performed under sedation as with the endoscopy. This test permits visualization of the bile ducts to determine whether there is any obstruction.

Gallstone: Hard mass composed of bile pigments, cholesterol and calcium salts that can form in the gall bladder.

Hepatic: refers to the liver.

Hepatic vein: one of the several short veins originating within the lobes of the liver as small branches, which unite to form the hepatic veins.

Hepato-renal syndrome: A type of Kidney (renal) failure associated with a number of liver disorders.

Hepatitis: An inflammation of the liver caused by viruses, toxic, substances or immunological abnormalities.

HAV: Hepatitis A virus.

HBV: Hepatitis B virus.

HCV: Hepatitis C virus.

Hida Scan: A series of scans of the abdomen performed to examine the bile draining out of the liver.

Immunology: The study of the human immune

system and all of the phenomena that are connected with the defence mechanisms of the body.

Immune System: The organs that are responsible for immunity. The primary lymphoid organs are the thymus and the bone marrow. The secondary lymphoid organs are the lymph nodes and lymphoid aggregates (spleen, tonsils, gastrointestinal lymph tissue and peyer's patches).

Immunity: The body's ability to resist infection, afforded by the presence of circulating antibodies and white cells.

Immunosuppressive medication: a drug that reduces the body resistance to infection and other foreign bodies by suppressing the body's immunity. Because the immunity is lowered during treatment with immunosuppressive, there is an increased susceptibility to infection and certain types of cancer.

Jaundice: A yellowing of the skin or whites of the eyes, indicating excess bilirubin (a bile pigment) in the blood.

Liver Biopsy: A liver biopsy is the removal of a small sample of liver tissue for examination under a microscope. It is performed to determine the extent of any damage in the liver or in any other part of the body. It helps in the diagnosis of the disease and it is carried out with a special hallow needle, inserted into the liver or other organ.

Nifedipine (Adalat): A drug used for treatment of blood pressure.

Nausea: The feeling that one is about to vomit

NMR Scan: Medical examination similar to a CT scan except that it uses magnetic resonance instead of X-ray

Osteoporosis: A disease that causes a loss of bone tissue resulting in bones to become brittle, fragile and liable to fracture. There are many reasons for osteoporosis, among them infection and injury. It is also a feature of cushing's disease and prolonged steroid drug.

Primary Biliary Cirrhosis, (PBC): A slow chronic liver disease that can gradually destroy the bile ducts within the liver, so that bile cannot be efficiently secreted.

Propranolol: A drug used to treat abnormal heart rhythm, angina, and high blood pressure and also taken to relieve anxiety.

Prednisolone: It is a steroid drug used to block some of the cells that trigger a rejection response. It is used immediately after the transplant in conjunction with other immunosuppressive (anti-rejection) medications.

Ranitidine (zantac): A drug to prevent irritation which may occur with stress as a side-effect of taking anti-rejection drug.

Renal: refers to the kidney

Tacrolimus FK 506, (Prograf): It is a powerful immunosuppressive drug, (anti-Rejection) used to prevent rejection of transplanted organs.

Transplantation: The implantation of an organ or a tissue from one part of the body to another, or from one person (the donor) to another (the recipient). See also xenotransplantation

Ultrasound: Medical test uses sound waves to create a picture of the liver and the surrounding organs. It may also be used to assess blood flow to and from the liver.

UKTS: UNITED Kingdom Transplant Service in Bristol.

Xenotransplantation: the transplantation of organs from one person to another. Research into the feasibility of transplanting pig organs into human body is under way.

Your liver is a vital organ look after it !

References

** Dr. A. Burroughs
   Towards Transplantation
** Dr. D. Patch
   Complications of Liver Disease
** Mr. K. Rolles
   Liver Transplantation
** Dr. J. Dooley
   Liver Imaging
** Prof. N. McIntyre
   Living With Liver Disease
** Prof. Jacques Cinqualbre
   Symbolism of the liver through the ages
** Linda Selves & Debbie Marshal
   Liver Transplantation
   Life After A Transplant
** American Liver Foundation Papers
** Australian liver foundation Papers
** British Liver Foundation Papers
** Canadian Liver Foundation Papers
** Euroliver Foundation Papers
** Hepatitis Foundation International Papers
** International Liver Transplantation Papers
** World Health Organization (WHO) Reports